THE ESSENTIAL PARISH NURSE

Dedication
For Steve, Sophia, and John,
the parish nurses and clergy in health ministry,
and the Deaconess Sisters

The Pilgrim Press, 700 Prospect Avenue East, Cleveland, Ohio 44115-1100
pilgrimpress.com
© 2003 by Deborah L. Patterson

Scripture quotations, unless otherwise noted, are from the *New Revised Standard Version of the Bible*, © 1989 by the Division of Christian Education of the National Council of Churches of Christ in the United States of America and are used by permission. Changes have been made for inclusivity.

Printed in the United States of America on acid-free paper

14   13   9   8   7

Library of Congress Cataloging-in-Publication Data

Patterson, Deborah L., 1956-
     The essential parish nurse : ABCs for congregational health ministry / Deborah L.
     Patterson; contributors, Mary Ann Brischetto ... [et al].
          p.   cm.
     Includes bibliographical references (p.).
     ISBN 0-8298-1571-6 (pbk. : alk. paper)
     1. Parish nursing.   I. Title.
RT120.P37P385   2003
610.73'43—dc22

                                                            2003066435

Contents

Foreword

PARISH NURSING, WE HAVE FOUND, is the most exciting and fulfilling of the nursing specialties. It is a dynamic process of working with parishioners and families in the community toward wholeness of body, mind, and spirit. Rev. Dr. Granger Westberg, a founder of modern parish nursing, stated that a nurse has the sensitivity—the peripheral vision, he called it—to see beyond the patient's problems and verbal statements. A nurse, he suggested, hears things that were left unsaid by the patient. Rev. Westberg believed that nurses seemed to be grounded both in the sciences and in the humanities, and were comfortable with both spiritual and physical natures.

Nursing is more than a profession—it is a passionate way of actively sharing God's unconditional love for all people through nursing education and care. Parish nursing is even more: it is nursing that is guided by the Holy Spirit, as the patient (parishioner or member of the community), the pastor, and the parish nurse journey together toward God within the context of the congregation and wider community.

Important truths are often difficult to share without a story. Therefore, we will share a couple of stories from our own experience. The first story is about a young adult, Roy, and his family.[1]

Roy moved back into his father's house, which is located near the church. A few weeks later, some windows on the third floor of the educational building were shattered. The neighborhood sources accused Roy. The parish nurse, Mary Ann, decided to make a home visit to assess the situation.

Mary Ann noted, "The door opened slowly. It took awhile for my eyes to adjust to the darkness inside the house. Both Roy's dad and his stepmother were blind. Roy's dad immediately became very defensive because they were aware of the neighborhood accusation."

"They are always out after Roy," his father said. Mary Ann requested Roy's help to clean up the glass and assured Roy and his Dad that Roy's help did not indicate any guilt—she simply needed help to clean up the mess. "It is through our actions of modeling compassion and God's unconditional love that the community may come to realize that our church can be a safe place where no judgment of always being wrong is made. Together we walked to the church and cleaned up the glass."

Mary Ann learned that throughout Roy's school years he had been the victim of many beatings and had dropped out of school at age sixteen. Since Roy was unable to achieve success through positive behavior, he received attention with negative behavior. After Roy and Mary Ann finished cleaning up the glass, they headed to the parish nurse office to discuss a mutually agreeable plan to continue with some positive social interactions. Roy had decided that the ultimate way to prove his importance to society was to be arrested. "You can even call my mom," Roy said with tears in his eyes, "she can tell you how bad I really am." Mary Ann replied, "Roy, it is real simple; there is no such thing as a bad kid. Sometimes kids just make dumb choices." This exchange initiated a trusting relationship between Roy and Mary Ann.

Mary Ann continued, "During the next few months Roy and I began sharing lunch. We talked about the lifestyle choices he was making and what his options were. When Pastor Bob began his ministry at St. Paul, he joined us for our luncheon rap sessions. Roy has now expanded his boundaries of trust to include Bob. The relationship that has been established gives Roy and his family the opportunity to make some positive lifestyle choices. As a result, Devon, Roy's nephew, attended the one-week Vacation Bible Experience at the church, Roy's parents received in-home doctor's care, and Roy is employed. The church has also benefited. Roy's family has given the church a ministry opportunity for an active outreach of God's love into the community."

The second story is about the incredible journey that Bob and Mary Ann took together with a parishioner toward the ultimate wholeness in God. The story began when one parishioner made a referral for another—her dear friend, Etta—to Mary Ann. An initial home visit with Etta was arranged with her friend present. During the visit Etta shared her past medical history and surgical intervention for her terminal illness. She also expressed her frustration with her past medical care. Mary Ann suggested, "Why don't you seek a second opinion?"

Etta was a little hesitant. Mary Ann, an experienced nurse, expressed her conviction about advocating for patients' rights, "As long as you reimburse the physician and he isn't reimbursing you, it is your right to seek a second opinion!" Acknowledging that four ears were better than two, Etta and Mary Ann headed to the new physician with the old medical data available.

After a comprehensive exam, the physician, being unsure of Etta's emotional status, informed Mary Ann of the terminal nature of his physical findings while Etta was dressing. Being familiar with Etta, Mary Ann assured the physician that she desired an honest and direct evaluation of her condition and her options. As they were leaving the physician's office, Etta turned to Mary Ann with tears in her eyes and said in a voice filled with remorse, "I wish we had gone to him first. I now understand what other treatments might have done for me after my surgery two years ago."

During the drive home Mary Ann made a suggestion to Etta, "I think it would be a good idea that Pastor Bob is made aware of your condition." Etta agreed that Bob should become involved in her care. At this time she did not yet wish for the congregation to be made aware of the situation. Bob and Mary Ann initiated a holistic plan, based on the physician's physical findings and Etta's spiritual needs. The interventions included home visitation by Bob and Mary Ann as needed, either individually or jointly. Initially, the visits had specific outcomes, such as reviewing her living will, carefully explaining and reviewing her wishes for the DNR (do not resuscitate) form, and contacting Hospice. A true and meaningful relationship began to develop between Etta, Bob, and Mary Ann.

Well, Etta surprised us! She did not experience the rapidly progressing prognosis initially given to her by the doctor. Bob and Mary Ann reevaluated their plan as Etta was able to maintain her normal activities, which included attending worship and caring for a friend who was recovering from surgery. The additional time granted to Etta allowed our visitations to lead to a close and trusting relationship. Etta was teaching Bob and Mary Ann the type of luggage that she needed to complete her wholistic journey, that is, what Etta needed to complete her time on earth and feel safe to die. It gave us time to learn of Etta's sorrows and of her joys, such as the tremendous relationship she and her dad shared, and her love of Christmas.

Etta had always looked forward to Christmas Eve and singing the first verse of "Silent Night" in her native German tongue. When Christmas Eve arrived this year the only light in the church came from the small white candles held by each member. Etta joined the choir in the front of the sanctuary to lead the hymn. Bob put his arm around Etta, a lump in his throat and tears in his eyes, as the choir started to sing. Bob and Etta knew that this was the last time that they would sing "Silent Night" together. What an emotional moment in the journey!

February arrived. It was cold and gloomy on our next jointly scheduled visit. Etta greeted us at the door, wrapped up in a blanket and appearing pale and anxious. Upon entering the living room, we had a sense that Etta had a purpose for our visit. Before we sat down, Etta turned toward Mary Ann and stated, "I need to talk to you privately." She and Mary Ann headed to the bathroom and addressed her concerns. As we suspected, the terminal phase of her illness was now progressing more rapidly. When we were back in the living room our conversation centered around Etta's wishes to be able to die at home. Her fear was not of death but of being alone and of her possible inability to handle the pain.

Even though she was getting physically weaker, she embodied an inner strength. We assured her that her wishes would be met. When Mary Ann left to purchase the needed supplies, Bob asked Etta, "What brings you peace during these days?" She showed him her prayer book and devotional material. She reminded Bob of her favorite hymns and scripture passages, which together they had considered on an earlier visit, while planning her funeral service. Etta was teaching us how she was dying with dignity.

We hope that through this book, pastors and interested lay leaders will be introduced to the concept of parish nursing in a way that will clearly demonstrate its importance to the outreach and evangelism ministry of a congregation, in partnership with clergy and lay volunteers.

Rev. Robert Keller, pastor
St. Paul United Church of Christ
St. Louis, Missouri

Mary Ann Brischetto, R.N., B.S.N., parish nurse
St. Paul United Church of Christ
St. Louis, Missouri

Preface and Acknowledgements

A NUMBER OF EXCELLENT RESOURCES ON parish nursing are available, from an early theological and practical treatise on parish nursing by Rev. Dr. Granger Westberg, who was the catalyst behind the modern parish nurse movement, which began in Chicago in the mid-1980s, to a comprehensive book for parish nurses edited by Phyllis Ann Solari-Twadell and Mary Ann McDermott, to a book on starting a health cabinet or wellness committee in churches by Jill Westberg McNamara. In addition, a new book by Verna Benner Carson and Harold G. Koenig has done much to popularize the parish nursing movement.[1] I highly recommend each of them to you for your further reading.

As interest in parish nursing continues to grow, however, coordinators of parish nurse programs increasingly are being called on to interpret to congregations the "ABCs" of developing a parish nurse program at this time. It is to fill this need that this book is designed.

My own interest in parish nursing springs from my years as a parish pastor. Most of the parishioners upon whom I called had health-related issues. I often wished that I had a colleague in ministry with expertise in health issues with whom I could confer and to whom I might refer parishioners and neighbors with health concerns.

I recall one parishioner taking what she called "nerve pills," who had undiagnosed breast cancer, and who, I am grateful to recall, took my advice for a second opinion and is still alive today. Was it the role of a pastor to suggest a second opinion? Certainly! A parish nurse, however, may have an even stronger drive for patient advocacy, since it would be one specific focus of her or his ministry.[2]

I recall another man who was sent home from the hospital to an empty house following surgery, with instructions for care that required assistance from others. The church was able to fill the breach, but it would have been so much easier to coordinate the needed services with a parish nurse who could arrange for quality home health care and assemble a care team of prepared volunteers.

I recall a parishioner with a mental illness that I did not understand and whose family did not know whether she was receiving adequate care. For this, and for a hundred other situations, I wish I had had a parish nurse as a colleague in ministry.

It was my very good fortune to be able to return to school following my tenure at that parish, through a scholarship provided by three church-related bodies: the Council for Health and Human Service Ministries of the United Church of Christ, Deaconess Health System in St. Louis, and Advocate Health Care in Chicago. I studied health administration at Washington University School of Medicine in St. Louis and soon began work at Deaconess Health System as Minister of Religion and Health. In that capacity, I oversaw the areas of Spiritual Care, Mission, Diakonal Ministry, and the department of Parish Nursing, which was headed by Alvyne Rethemeyer.

In 1997, the Board of Trustees of Deaconess Incarnate Word Health System decided not to compete for paying patients, but to return to the church's earlier vision of faith and health by selling the health system and converting the assets into funds to be used to improve the health of the St. Louis metropolitan community. The funds were distributed to two foundations, Deaconess Foundation and the Incarnate Word Foundation. At the time of the sale, the Parish Nurse Program was the one programmatic asset retained by the Deaconess Foundation because it was so closely related to the church's health-related outreach mission. At that time, the Parish Nurse Program had eight parish nurses on staff and a full-time coordinator. Recently, Deaconess Parish Nurse Ministries became separately incorporated, and on 1 January, 2002, it became home to the International Parish Nurse Resource Center, formerly located at Advocate Health Care in Chicago.

The Rev. Dr. Richard Ellerbrake, president emeritus of Deaconess Health System in St. Louis, has long referred to our health-care system as an "illness care system" and expounded that view in a keynote address at the 2002 Westberg Parish Nurse Symposium.[3] It is a point of view shared by the president and CEO of the Deaconess Foundation, Rev. Jerry W. Paul. Because of their commitment to the improved health of the community, the Deaconess Foundation and many other health foundations focus on wellness and prevention, rather than on acute care, and we are grateful for their continuing support to parish nursing in this region.

Parish nursing fits the model of wellness and prevention in a way that touches lives across generational, cultural, and socioeconomic lines. It draws a healing circle around a congregation and extends that circle into the community, blowing open the doors of churches in renewing and life-affirming ways. Once a congregation fully grasps the implications for change, healing, and hope inherent in the parish nursing model, it is forever changed.

It has been my privilege for many years to work with Alvyne Rethemeyer, the former director of Parish Nursing at Deaconess Parish Nurse Ministries and current director of the International Parish Nurse Resource Center, in the growth and development of parish nursing in the St. Louis metropolitan area. Much of her wisdom has gone into the development of this book. Ms. Rethemeyer is also responsible for the development of many of the resources found in the appendices, as well as for contributing chapter 13, "Now What? Helping a New Parish Nurse Get Started." Rev. Robert Keller and Mary Ann Brischetto, who work together as a pastor and parish nurse at St. Paul United Church of Christ in St. Louis, have contributed a helpful foreword and an outstanding chapter on working together as a team. Rev. Keller also serves on the board of the International Parish Nurse Resource Center. Elizabeth Durban, a Deaconess parish nurse at St. Gabriel's Catholic Church, an active and vital parish in the city of St. Louis, with a great track record of outstanding health fairs, has contributed the chapter on that topic.

I am also grateful to the Rev. Jerry W. Paul, president and CEO of the Deaconess Foundation, Norella Huggins, chair of the Board of Managers of Deaconess Parish Nurse Ministries, Rev. Dr. Richard Ellerbrake, president emeritus of Deaconess Health System (and officer of Deaconess Parish Nurse Ministries), Jill Westberg

McNamara, an early lay leader and author in the parish nursing movement, and Dr. Jane Westberg, who is writing her father's biography, for sharing their insights and providing editorial assistance with this book. Rev. Dr. Tom Tupper, vice president of the Deaconess Foundation, provided a great deal of assistance with the chapter on benefits for parish nurses. Finally, I would be remiss if I did not thank our office manager, Carolyn Loeffler, who helped gather the appendices and did a spectacular job of proofreading the entire manuscript.

In addition, I would like to thank those at Pilgrim Press, particularly Kim Sadler, Aimée Jannsohn, Kristin Firth, and Madrid Tramble for all their assistance with this book.

As we continue the work of Deaconess Parish Nurse Ministries and the International Parish Nurse Resource Center, we look forward to working with others in the fields of parish nursing and health ministries. We hope this book is helpful to you as you consider the option of parish nursing as one form of health ministry in your congregation.

For the many parish nurses I have been privileged to know, and for the many parish nurses and other health professionals from around the United States and from as far away as Korea and New Zealand that I have met through my work at the International Parish Nurse Resource Center, I am truly grateful. It is to these professionals, and to the clergy with whom they so diligently work, that this book is dedicated. It is to the clergy and nursing professionals considering this form of ministry that this book is addressed.

Blessings.

The Case for Parish Nursing as a Ministry of the Church

The Mandate to Heal and Its Expression in the Church

W HEN JESUS SENT OUT HIS disciples, he gave them a mandate to preach, teach, and heal. Over the centuries, the church has been doing very well with preaching—two thousand years after Jesus walked this earth, most Christian communities have preaching as a regular part of worship. The church has also been doing well with teaching—most congregations have active and vital Christian education programs. The church has never quite made up its mind, however, about where it wants to stand regarding Jesus' commission to heal.

The early church certainly embraced Jesus' instruction, especially through such actions as anointing with oil for healing (see James 5:13–16). The prevalent Mediterranean worldview during the first century, which was also shared by Jesus, held that disease either was caused by demons or was a punishment from God for sin (either of the person with the disease or of an ancestor, visited upon another generation).

The beginnings of modern medicine come to us through ancient Greece, with Hippocrates (born 460 B.C.E.) the most famous of its early physicians. As Roman rule spread, Greek medical schools were absorbed into that empire, and they then came under the influence of the Christian Church in later centuries. As it became more and more obvious to the Western world that there were scientific explanations for diseases and their treatments, the Church recoiled from medical science with fear that God would not be needed to heal.

The Church went back and forth between embracing medical care and condemning it. During the Middle Ages, many religious orders sprang up that devoted themselves to caring for the sick. Religious groups started most of the earliest hospitals around the world, and nearly all the present hospitals in America. At other periods in history, however, the Church was ambivalent toward or even actively opposed to Western medicine, as it was to other advances of science. Hostility reached extremes, such as closing medical schools in Athens and Alexandria in the sixth century, the papal edict of 1163 forbidding the clergy to shed blood in the performance of operations,[1] and later discouraging the seeking of medical treatment, which was seen as having a lack of faith in God's healing power.[2] Anointing with oil became a sacrament for the dying in the twelfth century, and the church's role in healing was relegated to the healing of souls only.

Many monastic orders were disbanded during the Reformation, and the institutions they ran, including hospitals, were closed. In England alone, it is estimated that over one hundred hospitals staffed by nuns were closed.[3] However, Protestant reformers such as Calvin also founded hospitals and took responsibility for the social welfare of the community.

In the mid-1800s, the Church became involved in a renaissance of assistance to the ailing that took expression in many forms. Let's take a look at the birth of one such example in America to explore how that vision was expressed.

A Church Responds to a Hurting Community

The Deaconess Sisterhood in St. Louis, Missouri, was started by a group of German Evangelical clergy and laity, both men and women, in 1889.[4] They had known about a model of health ministry begun in Kaiserswerth, Germany, by Rev. Theodore Fliedner and his wife, Frederike. The Fliedners established the modern "Deaconess" movement, in which women were trained as nurses representing the Church in service to the wider community. This movement has its origins in the first century Christian church, with deaconesses such as Phoebe.[5]

Begun in Kaiserswerth in 1836 with one young woman, the Deaconess movement grew to over 25,000 women serving in Europe, the United States, Egypt, Russia, India, and Hong Kong by the turn of the century. The education of Deaconesses was an important root of the professional practice of nursing. Even Florence Nightingale studied with the Fliedners in 1851 before beginning her work in the Crimean War and establishing the first nursing schools in England. In this way, the Church had a tremendous impact on the emergence of nursing as a profession.[6]

The Deaconess movement was also pivotal in the reconnection of service to others as a recognized ministry (diakonal ministry) within the church. This topic will be explored in greater detail in the following chapter.

One of the outposts of the Evangelical Deaconess movement in Germany appeared in St. Louis, Missouri, in 1889, when the Evangelical Church recruited two nurses who had been trained in Deaconess methods. Mrs. Katherine Haack and her niece, Lydia Daries, were consecrated on Sunday, 18 August 1889, as the first Evangelical Deaconess Sisters in St. Louis.[7]

The first health-care facility run by Sister Katherine and Sister Lydia was in their private home, a house purchased for the Sisters and donated to them in 1889 by Mrs. Dorothea Zipf.[8] Funds in the amount of two dollars per person annually were solicited from women's fellowships and from other church members. This facility, known as the Evangelische Diakonissenhaus (Evangelical Deaconess Home) began operations in St. Louis with the two Deaconesses and two house physicians who joined the staff a month later. One Deaconess worked in the home and one provided home care, each charging fifty cents per twenty-four-hour period.

At this time, St. Louis was the fourth largest city in the United States. In 1889 the city had much to boast about, such as widespread employment opportunities, fine schools and cultural institutions, and excellent public transportation. However, it also faced many challenges. Housing was often substandard, there were few social services available to help the poor, and the sanitation system left a great deal to be desired.[9] Diseases such as smallpox, polio, and tuberculosis were dreaded and common.

In the late nineteenth century, the sick and injured were cared for at home whenever possible, and only the destitute or medically desperate would be cared for in a hospital. Most surgeries were performed at home. The life expectancy for a rural American around

1890 was only about forty years and was even lower for city dwellers. Hospitals were disparagingly called "pest houses" because the poor were cared for there, and hospital caregivers often had less than outstanding backgrounds. No one wanted the poor "in their backyard." For this reason churches decided to step into the breach.

Only patients who could not be taken care of in their own homes (where Deaconesses sometimes went to live and help with managing the entire household, provide child care, cook and clean, as well as care for the ill family member) went to stay in the Deaconess Home where the Sisters lived. At the beginning the home was called "Deaconess Home" and only later became the "Deaconess Home and Hospital."

In the Deaconess Home and Hospital, meals prepared by women in the churches augmented the food served to the patients, and congregational volunteers helped with some routine patient care. Drugs and vaccines that we take for granted today, including antibiotics, were unknown, and diagnostic technology, including x-ray, was in its infancy. The congregational volunteer in 1889 could provide health care that was nearly on a par with the trained professional.

The costs for health-care services in 1889 were minimal as well. It is interesting to note that, at the turn of the century, the salary for a physician was the same as a clergy salary. In fact, surgeons would occasionally give haircuts to supplement their income. Health insurance was unknown by the general public, although some plans were beginning to appear around the turn of the century. Not until after World War II would a large part of the U.S. population have health insurance.

In 1889, the cost for staying in the Deaconess Home and Hospital was five dollars per week, payable in cash at admission, with any remainder to be returned upon discharge. Confinements for labor and delivery of a child generally lasted several weeks, and the hospital administrator, an Evangelical clergyman, performed many baptisms during that time. In fact, the average length of stay for all hospitalizations was around forty days, which, twenty-five years later, had decreased to "only" twenty-six days.

Fast forward to today. Labor and delivery in an American hospital will "confine" a woman only for a day or two. Much surgery is done on an outpatient basis. Consider the removal of cataracts, previously performed by a surgeon using a scalpel in a hospital, with the patient remaining hospitalized with his or her head immobilized by sandbags for days. Now, cataract removal is performed on an outpatient basis using laser technology, and the patient is only detained a few hours.

Deaconess was located in an urban neighborhood by the late twentieth century, having made an earlier decision to remain in the city of St. Louis rather than to move to the rapidly expanding suburbs. It was a community hospital, with a college of nursing, and provided a great deal of care to the poor and uninsured. By the 1990s Deaconess had expanded many times, acquired other hospitals, and finally merged with Incarnate Word Hospital. In 1997, because Deaconess Incarnate Word Health System questioned whether competing for paying patients was the best use of its church-related resources in a metro area with an excess number of hospital beds among the highest in the nation, the decision was made to sell the health system assets and to use the proceeds to improve the health of the St. Louis metropolitan area in other ways, such as through parish nursing and through grants to improve children's health in the region.[10]

So, does there remain a role for the church to play in healing in these days of lasers and ultrasound? The love/hate relationship between the church and the scientific/medical community over the centuries with regard to healing has not yet been reconciled. Churches stay away from the issue of physical health, believing that healing belongs only to the purview of trained medical professionals as well as not wanting to walk into the waters of "faith healing." The medical community looks with great suspicion on "outsiders" who have not gone through the rigorous training required at medical schools, yet who feel they deserve a role and voice in health care.

I believe that the church does have a profound role to play in health care and an important and necessary voice that must be heard. Health ministry, along with preaching and teaching, is the church's mandate from its rock and cornerstone, Jesus the Living and Healing Christ. It is not an optional ministry—it is an integral part of the Church's calling. The question becomes—how is the Church going to live out and fulfill its health ministry? Parish nursing is one vital way to have an effective health ministry in a faith community.

A Closer Look at Parish Nursing as a Health Ministry of the Church

Certainly much has changed in our understanding of the cause of disease and treatment of illness since Jesus' day. Much has also changed in the way we live. We live in a society that is increasingly long-lived and increasingly mobile, with many adults living far from their nuclear and/or extended families. Isolation is a serious issue for many elderly parents with health concerns whose children have moved to another part of the country, or for couples raising their children far from other family members. These people often look to the church for help and support.

Economic pressures are also major stressors, especially when families are without any or adequate health insurance, are without access to needed services, and are at risk of falling through the cracks should illness strike them. Currently, more then forty-one million Americans lack health insurance coverage. In 2002, 1.4 million joined the ranks of the medically uninsured, and the largest group (about eight hundred thousand) of that number was among people who had incomes in excess of $75,000. They either lost their jobs or found themselves priced out of the health-care market by steeply rising health insurance premiums.[11]

Americans face a surfeit of competing challenges within the health arena: health information is available everywhere from the Internet to magazines, to racks of brochures at the grocery store, yet we do not have enough personal attention from health professionals to help us know which of it is applicable, or even accurate. Under managed care, physicians are under pressure to see patients quickly—some must schedule appointments as short as seven minutes per patient. Many people need help to discover options for needed services, to advocate for themselves, and even to understand their diagnoses or their health risks.

We live in a society that encourages a sedentary lifestyle—television and computers keep us sitting and still. Our diets are too often filled with salt, fat, and sugar. We are sleep-deprived and we drive too fast.

So what are the health issues that a parish nurse can address in a congregation? Education about wellness and attention to the care of physical illness is at the top of the list, of course. A parish nurse has time to spend with individuals to help them look at their lifestyles and understand their health risks or to explain a diagnosis or treatment of illness. Mental illness strikes many families in our churches, as in the wider population, and these members must be welcomed and supported. A parish nurse can arrange for educational programs to help a faith community understand mental health issues and ways to support the mentally ill person and his or her family members. Alcohol and drug abuse, domestic violence, sexual abuse, and random violence are also factors that impact many church members and neighbors, and that cause great shame. Many in our society feel isolated and lonely, leading health risk factors. The parish nurse can work with a congregation to develop responses to these issues or proactive prevention programs. The church must be equipped to help people toward wholeness of body, mind, spirit, and community, and a parish nurse can play an important role in equipping the church for that mission.

A new parish nurse generally finds that individuals seek her or him out in this order: the isolated elderly, middle-aged men with health concerns, parents of teenagers with parenting questions, parents of young children who are concerned about their children's health and development, and then many others in the congregation. A parish nurse is able to provide help in all these areas, and more.

I believe that a parish nurse can be an essential part of health ministry in any congregation, whether it is in an inner city, an outer suburb, or a rural community. The economics of the congregation and its membership should not argue against a parish nurse. Relatively well-to-do church members may not see the need for such a ministry in their congregation because they have the financial resources to acquire any needed services. Financially strapped congregations may feel that they can't afford such a ministry. However, I firmly believe that health ministry is for all, just as preaching and teaching is for all. We all need to be healthy and whole.

If a congregation wishes to respond to Christ's command to heal as well as to preach and teach, it needs to take seriously the work of health ministry. Parish nursing is a vital and effective ministry, which can make a significant impact on the health of a community in many critical ways.

In the final analysis, God is life giving, and the Church is called to share Christ's ministry of calling God's people to wholeness. We are called to preach, teach, and heal—to bring hope for healing and well being for the whole people of God as spiritual, emotional, intellectual, physical, and social beings.

Sacred Footsteps

Diakonal Ministry and
Its Relationship to Parish Nursing

*D*IAKONIA IS THE GREEK WORD for "service." Early in the development of the Christian church, service on behalf of the Church to the community was identified as needing to be a recognized ministry. This form of ministry (as opposed to preaching sermons or teaching classes to those who wished to join the Church) became known as "diakonal ministry."

Diakonal ministry can be either the action performed, or an official role in the church. In Acts 6, we read of the diakonal ministry of table-service, which allowed other leaders in the church to engage in ministries of preaching and teaching. In this example, the disciples chose Stephen (hence the popular name for a form of diakonal ministry known as "Stephen Ministry") and a number of others. The apostles then prayed and laid their hands on these new ministers serving the church.

"Offices" (deacons and deaconesses) for service ministry were also held by men and women in the early church, such as seen in Romans 16:1–2, where Paul writes, "I commend to you our sister Phoebe, a deaconess of the church in Cenchrea. I ask you to receive her in the Lord in a way worthy of the saints and to give her any help she may need from you, for she has been a great help to many people, including me (NIV)." Diakonal ministry as an office reappears in very stylized form after the Reformation among the followers of John Calvin.

Diakonal ministry was a fusion of care for body and soul, done in the context of community, and tied to the roots of worship (*leitourgia* in Greek). Diakonal ministry was the responsibility both of the individual and of the community, not the isolated spiritual practice of one lone Christian. As Gary Gunderson, director of the Interfaith Health Program at Emory University has pointed out in today's context: "Spirituality doesn't make hospital calls."[1] Diakonal ministry was service done on behalf of the Church, in response to God's love, which had been shown through Jesus Christ to the person performing the service.

There are several theological frameworks for Christian *diakonia*, all of which are valid. The first is that when we do diakonal ministry, we follow the example set by Christ in serving those in need. A person operating out of this viewpoint would hold that since Jesus spent his life serving the sick and troubled, if we are Christians, we should have a similar kind of ministry.

Another viewpoint is seeing *diakonia* as an opportunity to serve as a witness for Christ. This is approaching service to others with the belief that if we are merciful and compassionate, we will draw others to salvation. Many of the medical missionaries who served during the eighteenth century in "foreign" countries held this viewpoint, which was also popular among Protestant missionary societies.

A third view maintains that in serving those in need, we provide service to Christ. This theology is very strong and was lived out through the works of Christians like Mother Teresa and Dorothy Day. In fact, in a famous prayer of Mother Teresa, she specifically prays to see Christ in each person to whom she ministers.

Diakonia was proclamation about God, about the Church, and about what it meant to be a Christian. This Christian ministry proclaimed that service to the poor and sick by the Church meant that God cared passionately about the poor, the sick, the widow, the orphan, as well as about those who seemed to "have it made." It proclaimed that the Christian community was called to share all things in common and to leave not even one of God's children behind. Finally, it proclaimed that each and every Christian was a part of the body of Christ, with unique gifts to be used in the service of others.[2]

Diakonia in the early Church was unusual among the religions of its day. Non-Christians were surprised that the Christians would care about the poor, sick, and dying. During the fourth century, Christians buried over ten thousand who died from the plague, using their own resources. At this time, they also began to organize hospitals and other social agencies to help the needy.[3] During the fifth through sixteenth centuries, monasticism and related institutions grew and spread.

In the sixteenth century, the Church split in what became known as the Reformation, partially because of a fundamental difference in the way diakonal ministry was understood. The Roman Catholics believed that it was acceptable to be poor, and that in giving alms one receives a blessing. The Protestant Reformation occurred shortly after the fall of feudalism and the rise of the merchant class, when most in Europe lived in great poverty. The opinion set forth by Martin Luther (1483–1546) was that it was a shame to have poor within a Christian community, and that the poor must be relieved in response to God's love, a belief that fueled many of his writings.

Luther preached that although we are saved by faith, works are a response to salvation, and that all Christians were called to God's holy work—hence, the "priesthood of all believers." For Luther, diakonal ministry was not an office, but a service done in response to God's love. He organized a Community Chest, with funds to pay for schools and care of the sick and abandoned.

John Calvin in Geneva, Switzerland (1509–1564), saw *diakonia* as an office and created four recognized offices in his church: presbyter (preacher), elder (teacher), male deacon (administrator), and female deaconess (hands-on service). Every adult in the church was assigned a function, and the church was to operate as the "hands of God," with the care of the poor and the sick as the obligation of the Church.

During the centuries that followed, many other leaders in Christian churches found ways to express ministry far beyond preaching or teaching about God's love through words. The health and human service ministries of August Hermann Francke (1663-1727) and of Theodore and Frederike Fliedner (1800s) in Germany; the prison ministry of Elizabeth Fry (1780–1845) in England; the educational, health, and agricultural outreach ministries of Jean-Frederic Oberlin (1740–1826) and his parish associate Louise Scheppler (1763–1837), who founded the first kindergartens in France; the social reform ministries of John Howard (1726–1790) and Robert Owen (1771–1858) in England are but a few examples. The stories of any of these faithful Christians are inspiring to any pastor, parish nurse, or other church member. Elizabeth Fry's diakonal ministry within the framework of the Quaker faith tradition illustrates this remarkable outreach well.

Imagine a woman with eleven children, born into a wealthy family, whose religious yearnings led her to care for women and their children in the prisons of England in the beginning of the nineteenth century, where cruelty, degradation, and neglect were the order of the day. Imagine her being the first woman other than the Queen called to testify before the English Parliament. Imagine her traveling around Europe, taking a public stand for the humane treatment of the mentally ill and for the abolition of slavery at a time when these were most unpopular causes. The diakonal ministry of Elizabeth Fry changed the world. Her legacy of faith in action on behalf of her faith community remains with us to this day.

The need for diakonal ministers has always been great: one nineteenth-century church in Berlin, for example, had 89,000 parishioners and only five pastors. Diakonal ministries were faith-based responses to human needs at a time when governments had no organized response, and the Church could not respond through the work of the ordained pastoral clergy alone.

Certainly, few congregations, if any, today have 89,000 members, yet few are so small that the pastor alone can address all needs. The diakonal ministry of parish nursing is needed now as much as ever. Parish nurses follow in the footsteps not only of Florence Nightingale, who single-handedly changed health care forever, but of the cloud of witnesses whose professions and passions were fused together to serve and witness to Christ through the relief and prevention of human suffering.

The Church must call forth health ministers and other diakonal ministers who are able to step out in faith and embrace their work as a call from God to the service of the Church and an outreach to the community. This work may take diakonal ministers to places of which they have never dreamed. Parish nurses, as diakonal ministers, are following sacred footsteps, doing Jesus' work, touching others, as John Calvin would say, "with the hands of God."

Forging a New Path

A Brief History of Parish Nursing

L IKE THE VISIONARIES IN THE nineteenth century, such as Oberlin and the Fliedners, who saw the possibilities for outreach ministry, Rev. Dr. Granger Westberg was a visionary for our time who saw how congregations could impact the health of their communities. As a young Lutheran pastor in Bloomington, Illinois, Rev. Westberg had an opportunity to fill in for a chaplain at Augustana Hospital in Chicago for a week—a week that, as he says, changed his life. At that time, most chaplains were elderly clergy who had no clinical pastoral education and worked only part-time. Typically they went from patient to patient, distributing devotional materials and offering a prayer. During his week at Augustana Hospital, Rev. Westberg was disappointed that most of the physicians and some of the nurses did not take the spiritual mission of the hospital very seriously. He was also convinced that chaplains needed skills in counseling and other health-related fields if they were to be regarded as competent members of the health-care team. In the months that followed his week at Augustana, Rev. Westberg began envisioning and writing about new, more meaningful roles for chaplains. He argued that competent, well-educated chaplains could help revitalize the church's hospital ministry.

Three years later, when Augustana Hospital needed a new chaplain, Rev. Westberg asked to be considered for the position. Since he was a young man with a promising future, most of his colleagues thought he was crazy. He had big dreams, though, so he persisted and got the job. In 1944 after participating in some clinical pastoral education programs, Rev. Westberg became the first full-time chaplain at Augustana.

One of Rev. Westberg's first innovations was the creation of a course on the religious aspects of illnesses, as part of the nursing curriculum. In those days most of the schools of nursing in Christian hospitals did not include this topic in their curricula. Among other things, Rev. Westberg had student nurses do verbatim write-ups of patient encounters, which they then discussed in class. He wrote and lectured about the nurse's unique and important contribution to the care of patients.

Rev. Westberg's innovations in the work of the chaplain, clinical pastoral education, the doctor-patient relationship, and the team approach to health care led to his appointment in 1952 as chaplain of the University of Chicago Clinics and associate professor of Pastoral Care in the Federated Theological Faculty. Four years later, following his creative work in religion and health, he was given appointments at the University of Chicago, both in the divinity school and the medical school. This made him the first person at a major university to have such a joint appointment. While at Chicago, Rev. Westberg advocated for and demonstrated "wholistic" approaches to health care. Convinced that more attention needed to be paid to preventing illness and reaching people in the first stages of illnesses, he also set up several community-based health-care programs involving ministers and physicians.

In 1964 as the first dean of the Institute of Religion at the Texas Medical Center in Houston, Rev. Westberg further explored the concept of the parish as a potentially healing community. Later, as professor of Practical Theology at Wittenberg University's Hamma School of Theology in Springfield, Ohio, he established a church clinic, with volunteer doctors, nurses, ministers, and seminary students. The church clinic in Ohio was in a poor, underserved neighborhood. While he was speaking at Howard Medical School in Washington, D.C., members of the audience challenged him to consider expanding that vision of church clinics to middle- and upper-class neighborhoods so that they would not acquire the stigma of being a form of health delivery only for the poor. While searching for support for what he was now calling "wholistic health centers," Rev. Westberg met with Dr. Edward Lichter, chair of the Department of Preventative Medicine and Community Health at the University of Illinois College of Medicine. Dr. Lichter gave Rev. Westberg an appointment in his department and together they secured funding from the W. K. Kellogg Foundation and set up more than a dozen "Wholistic Health Centers."

Here is what Rev. Dr. Granger Westberg had to say about why he and his colleagues chose to put Wholistic Health Centers in churches:

> Wholistic Health Centers are located in churches for a reason. We think better health care can be given in the setting of an institution dedicated to healthful living. The average doctor's office does not have the kind of space we have in churches where there are rooms devoted to youth, music, meditation and many rooms for continuing education classes and seminars. The intention of churches is to have an active program of learning for people of all ages. They want their members to be kept abreast of the latest thinking concerning one's faith and one's life.
>
> Many medical journal articles say that "the way a person looks at life affects his health." Good health care then requires a more wholistic approach to the many facets of a person's being related to his illness or health. Our patients need to be engaged in many different kinds of health giving experiences—particularly in support groups where they meet people who can enrich their lives, give more meaning to daily living.
>
> We must learn how to utilize the rich human resources to be found in every congregation, many of which can be put to use for the upbuilding of people who are in need of the extra lift from a fellow human. Our Centers will be more wholistic to the degree they integrate all of their healing talent with the community of faith, which is the people of a worshipping congregation who deep down in their heart would like to find avenues of expression for the gratitude they feel to God.[1]

In these experimental settings, which became teaching centers for many doctors, nurses, and pastors from the United States and abroad, it became clear that the catalyst in the relationship between faith and health were the nurses. Rev. Westberg observed that the nurses "seemed to have one foot in the sciences and thereby were able to bridge the unnecessary gap between these two very old and esteemed professions."[2]

In 1979, Rev. Westberg edited a publication entitled *Theological Roots of Wholistic Health Care*, which contained essays by theologians and other ministry professionals involved with the Wholistic Health Centers. One very helpful piece in that volume is "The Religious Roots of Wholistic Health Care" by Thomas A. Droege, then professor at Valparaiso University, later to become the first director of the Interfaith Health Program at the Carter Center (now at Emory University).

Unfortunately, it was soon clear that the cost of financing clinics in churches was prohibitively expensive for most congregations, so Rev. Westberg considered a model using nurses whom he called "parish nurses" as the bridge between the Church and modern medicine.

In 1979, the first Health Cabinet was formed within a congregation at Community of Christ the Servant Church in Lombard, Illinois, to explore health ministry and the form it could take within that congregation. A book entitled *The Health Cabinet: How to Start a Wellness Committee in Your Church* was written by Jill Westberg McNamara, a member of that congregation, in 1981, documenting that journey and outlining the theological background and logistics developed by that congregation.[3] The Health Cabinet became an important component in the development of a parish nurse program within a congregation.

Lutheran General Hospital and Evangelical Health System, which merged in 1995 to form Advocate Health Care in Chicago, were committed to financially supporting the experimental parish nurse program and began to place paid parish nurses in congregations around the Chicago metropolitan area, primarily in Lutheran and United Church of Christ congregations. Their program has since grown to nearly thirty parish nurses.

Lutheran General was also committed to the growth and development of parish nursing elsewhere, so in 1985, the hospital created the Parish Nurse Resource Center (later to become the International Parish Nurse Resource Center, or IPNRC). Under the direction of Ann Solari-Twadell, the IPNRC grew rapidly to provide support and education for parish nursing, both in the United States and abroad. Shortly thereafter, Rev. Westberg and others began the Health Ministries Association as a membership organization for parish nurses and others interested in health ministry.

In 1986, the Parish Nurse Resource Center began to sponsor an annual professional meeting on parish nursing, called the Westberg Symposium. The symposium, named in honor of Rev. Dr. Granger Westberg, grew in attendance from eighty-four that first year to over eight hundred registrants in 2001.[4]

The Westberg Symposium was an arena in which the latest research and practice patterns in parish nursing could be presented. It also served as a gathering place to explore cutting-edge work in faith and health. The nurse association in the state in which the symposium was held awarded continuing education credits for the lectures and peer-reviewed paper presentations. The first fifteen years of the symposium were held in Chicago, and the sixteenth meeting was in St. Louis, Missouri. It is now sponsored by Deaconess Parish Nurse Ministries, which has been the home of the International Parish Nurse Resource Center since January of 2002. Deaconess Parish Nurse Ministries (DPNM) is located on the campus of Eden Theological Seminary in Webster Groves and is financially supported through the Deaconess Foundation.

In 1987, Rev. Dr. Westberg's and Jill Westberg McNamara's seminal work, *The Parish Nurse: Providing a Minister of Health for Your Congregation*, was published. This resource helped congregations understand Rev. Westberg's vision for parish nursing, which was beginning to take shape in Illinois, Iowa, Missouri, Wisconsin, and a few other areas around the United States.[5] At that time, there were only eight parish nurses as part of the parish nurse program at Lutheran General Hospital in Chicago.

The work of Rev. Westberg, Jill Westberg McNamara, Ann Solari-Twadell and others in Chicago put a name to what had been a movement of the Holy Spirit underway for quite some time. Nurses had been visiting parishioners in homes since the infancy of nursing. In fact, one can say that the entire nursing profession had been profoundly influenced by "parish nursing," given that Florence Nightingale, who is credited as being the founder of the nursing profession, had her sole nursing training at the church-related Deaconess school in Kaiserswerth, Germany, where the Fliedners had educated young church women to replicate the nursing care of the sick they saw being administered by the Mennonites in Holland. Rev. Westberg gave this rebirth of deaconess nursing the name "parish nursing," a title that was copyrighted by the International Parish Nurse Resource Center.

A number of registered nurses, such as Judy Teuscher, current parish nursing representative for the Missouri District of the Lutheran Church Missouri Synod, had been doing parish nursing since the 1960s. Judy would accompany her husband, a pastor, on home visits and was doing health assessment and intervention, as an integrator of faith and health, long before this form of ministry had a name and was recognized as a specialized practice of ministry by the American Nurses Association. Other nurses, such as Evangelical Deaconess Sister Bena Fuchs, had been doing this work before the First World War, relating to churches such as that connected with the Caroline Mission in St. Louis. Her diary is filled with stories of a wholistic approach to health care, including securing health-care access, arranging for referrals to other resources, coordinating volunteers, doing health-care assessment and intervention—indeed—her work included all the roles of the parish nurse of today! What is very old has become new again. It is perhaps a shame that there is a need for such a nursing specialty in today's medically advanced world, yet there will always be a need for wellness and for wholistic approaches to care within a faith community.

During the 1980s and 1990s, the International Parish Nurse Resource Center oversaw the development and review of an excellent parish nurse basic preparation curriculum, in consultation with expert faculty and parish nurse coordinators from around the country. This curriculum, called "Parish Nurse Basic Preparation," is a comprehensive set of lesson plans written by two dozen experienced parish nurse educators from institutions around the United States and abroad. Currently it is in use by more than eighty colleges, universities, and parish nurse programs around the country, known as "Educational Partners" with the IPNRC.

The International Parish Nurse Resource Center also developed two other classes that help to support the growth and development of parish nursing. The Parish Nurse Coordinator's Preparation class is designed for new parish nurse coordinators in various settings. The Faculty Preparation class is intended for parish nurse coordinators and nursing school faculty who wish to teach the Parish Nurse Basic Preparation curriculum in their universities or health systems.

In this way, the IPNRC provides consultation and support for the start-up of parish nurse ministries and programs in hundreds of hospitals and congregations around the country and abroad, and works with scores of colleges and universities in developing their educational programs for parish nursing.

Currently, approximately four thousand parish nurses have completed the parish nurse basic preparation class, and probably several thousand other parish nurses have attended other parish nurse classes. Many other registered nurses who have not yet attended such a class are working as parish nurses as well. There probably are close to ten thousand parish nurses in the United States and growing numbers in other countries around the world.[6]

Exact numbers of the parish nurses in America and abroad are not available, for a number of reasons. First of all, not all nurses who attend a parish nurse preparation class find a position as a parish nurse. Second, not all parish nurses have attended parish nurse basic preparation classes offered by an educational partner of the International Parish Nurse Resource Center. Finally, many volunteer parish nurses (some of whom have attended Parish Nurse Basic Preparation) should certainly be included in the total count of parish nurses who are serving congregations.

It must be stressed, however, that there is a very clear definition of the practice of parish nursing in the *Scope and Standards of Parish Nursing Practice*, as developed by the Health Ministries Association, in partnership with the American Nurses Association.[7] Not every nurse working with a congregation is doing so in the role of a parish nurse, and congregations are encouraged to review this document carefully in order to avoid liability exposure when putting together a parish nurse program.

Suffice it to say, parish nursing is growing rapidly. Parish nurse programs and networks now exist in almost every state and province of the United States and Canada, as well as many places abroad, especially Swaziland, Australia, and Korea. Interest in and research on parish nursing is exploding.

The most well-known leader of the modern day movement of parish nursing, Rev. Dr. Granger E. Westberg, then of Willowbrook, Illinois, died at age eighty-five on 16 February 1999 at Good Samaritan Hospital in Downer's Grove, Illinois. He was survived by his wife and ministry partner of almost sixty years, Helen, four children—Jane Westberg, John Westberg, Joan Onder, and Jill McNamara—eight grandchildren, and, at the time of this writing, one great-grandchild.

Parish nursing as envisioned by Rev. Westberg was a concept both old and innovative, forging a new path down a road trod by faithful clergy, laity, and nursing professionals a century earlier. Rev. Westberg gave the parish nursing movement a name and a strong theological underpinning, and he also had the amazing tenacity and vision to see parish nursing take hold throughout the United States and in other countries as well. We—clergy, parish nurses, and laity—would do well to follow in his remarkable footsteps to bring the world a little closer to healing and wholeness.

Not the Home Health Department
The Roles of a Parish Nurse

OFTEN, A GREAT DEAL OF confusion arises about what a parish nurse is expected to do. A parish nurse serves a number of roles in a local congregation and neighborhood. To understand these roles, it is helpful first to note what a parish nurse is *not*:

- A parish nurse is not a physician. He or she will not provide a medical diagnosis or medical treatment.

- A parish nurse is not a home health-care nurse. A parish nurse will not dispense medications or provide treatments prescribed by a physician.

- A parish nurse is not a therapist. She or he will not do physical therapy, occupational therapy, or psychotherapy.

- A parish nurse is not a clergyperson. A parish nurse usually does not hold a degree in theology, although many have some further education in theology or clinical pastoral education. All parish nurses come to the field with a deep spiritual commitment, and some are, in fact, ordained.

Varied Roles

The roles of a parish nurse generally include the following:

Integrator of faith and health. Health is not the absence of disease. Health is a holistic way of living that embraces life in its fullness, including the pursuit of a healthy spiritual life and connection to God and God's people. Often a parishioner feels a deep connection between a physical health concern and a spiritual concern. A parish nurse assists parishioners to achieve higher levels of wellness by improving both their spiritual and physical health.

Health educator. Health information surrounds us in this technological age. We have television, radio, the Internet, magazines, newspapers, even brochures in the grocery stores and billboards on the freeway. Interpreting this data for one's own health often requires a living, breathing health professional. Parish nurses are available to congregations for health education, and they provide opportunities for a congregation to learn about health issues, individually and in groups.

Health counselor. To whom do parishioners go with health concerns? Parishioners may already have been to physicians but may not fully understand a diagnosis or options for treatment. They may have medications that have expired, or that negatively interact with other medications (of which the physician may have been unaware). They may wonder if their health concerns even warrant seeing a doctor. A parish nurse is available to discuss health concerns, emphasizing early response to small problems and encouraging healthy lifestyle changes.

Referral advisor. Where does a parishioner go if he or she needs a second opinion, needs to find a nursing home or home health services for a loved one, or needs to find a counselor or other service? Parish nurses spend a great deal of time networking and investigating the quality of service providers in many different arenas of health care. A parish nurse in a congregation is available to provide referrals to health-care and social services within the community upon request from a parishioner.

Health advocate. Far too often, needed services are not available to an individual or even to large numbers of people in a given area. One example is the dearth of dental services available to the uninsured in the St. Louis area. Parish nurses here have been advocating for this service for years and are now working with other groups in St. Louis to make these services available. A parish nurse helps members of the congregation or community obtain needed health-related services.

Developer of support groups. A community often has needs for support groups, such as Alcoholics Anonymous, a grief support group, a weight loss support group, or a cancer survivors support group. A parish nurse is often familiar with the best programs and speakers in many of these areas. A parish nurse facilitates the development of support groups for the faith community and others served.

Volunteer coordinator. Many of the health-related needs of a congregational member, such as for transportation to the doctor or other medical appointments, for food during convalescence, or for child care during an illness, can be provided through volunteers. The parish nurse may work closely with "Faith in Action" groups[1] or with Volunteer Interfaith Caregivers. A parish nurse recruits, prepares and oversees congregational volunteers who help those in need.

A sample job description is included in appendix A of this book. Based on the Scope and Standards of Parish Nurse Practice, parish nurses are expected to serve in each of the roles just listed in order to fulfill their job description. Of course, an individual parish nurse's gifts and interests will influence where she or he is primarily drawn— perhaps more to health education and less to advocacy, or more to developing a strong volunteer network and less to developing support groups. However, a parish nurse must respond to the needs of a community as they are identified and not avoid the roles that are more difficult for him or her.

A parish nurse's specific assignments within the ministry of a congregation are decided in consultation with the pastor, other church leaders, and/or the parish nursing advisory committee or health cabinet in the parish. They may decide that the ministry should be primarily an outreach ministry to the surrounding neighborhood or a very specialized ministry, such as parish nursing within a school attached to a church. Most parishes, however, find that the parish nurse serves very broadly in response to the needs of the congregation. For a sample health needs survey, which can be used as tool to begin to identify some of the perceived health needs of a congregation or the community, please see appendix B.

You've Seen One Parish Nurse, You've Seen One Parish Nurse

The Role of the Health Cabinet

I MAGINE A CONGREGATION IN WHICH those who face surgery are routinely visited by a nurse, who helps explain the procedure and projected recovery. Imagine all expectant mothers being visited by a nurse who educates them about the importance of and access to prenatal care, and arranges a service of blessing before the child is born. Imagine a church where those who are ill and in need of support have meals, housekeeping, and transportation to appointments provided for them. Imagine a place where families who are looking for a nursing home get professional help in choosing, where members and neighbors are routinely screened for health concerns, where everybody is helped to access the health-care system. Imagine a church home where human beings receive care for body, mind, and spirit. Imagine a church that has recovered the idea of a geographical parish and cares for those living in the vicinity of the church, members and nonmembers alike. A congregation with a parish nurse ministry can be such a place. But how does it begin the task of starting such a ministry? This is the role of the health cabinet.

What is a Health Cabinet?

A health cabinet is composed of a small group of individuals, usually about five to seven in number, drawn from health professionals and others who are interested in exploring issues of faith and health in a congregational setting. Some churches prefer to call the health cabinet by other names—a health committee or health council, or something like "Caring Friends." The name is not that important, but the existence and action of such a group is critical. For ease of our discussion, we will use "health cabinet" here.[1]

A parish nurse ministry is generally first the idea of an individual or two within a congregation who has heard of the concept and would like to see it happen in their own setting. They generally talk with others in the congregation and with the pastor. (Of course, often the person who wants to start a parish nurse ministry is the pastor, so this step can be dispensed with!)

A health cabinet should be formed as soon as possible after the idea for health ministry comes up, to promote the greatest partnership in such a program over the long haul. It is a fact of human nature that people prefer to have ownership in an idea before they support it. Having a committee of people who had significant input into the creation and design of a parish nurse ministry proposal will go a long way toward making it of interest to the rest of the congregation. Those who are unfamiliar with parish nursing may think, erroneously, of a parish nurse as a "home health nurse" or a nurse to care only for the uninsured.

In addition, putting a health cabinet into place early in the process is critical because parish nursing is a ministry of the congregation, not of the individual performing the ministry. While stories of successful "lone wolf" type parish nurses abound, great difficulty is encountered in replacing that person should he or she no longer provide the service. Also, maintaining that same nurse when the pastoral leadership changes, without the support and ongoing commitment of a health cabinet working to grow and develop health ministry in the congregation and community, may be very difficult. A committee that has made a significant investment of time and energy into a program will want to see it grow and prosper over time.

It is important to remember that a parish nurse health ministry is not a "one-size-fits-all" endeavor in which a parish nurse is hired and set to work magically making all well. Alvyne Rethemeyer, director of the International Parish Nurse Resource Center, is often heard to say, "You have seen one parish nurse ministry, you have seen one parish nurse ministry." There are many different approaches to creating a parish nurse ministry, and one task of the health cabinet is to help the parish nurse in strategically planning and leading that congregation's health outreach. Let's take a closer look at the work of a health cabinet.

What Does a Health Cabinet Do?

The first task of a health cabinet is to learn as much as possible about the theological framework for developing a health ministry in a congregation. The health cabinet should also learn as much as possible about the field of parish nursing as one option for health ministry. Good resources for this include, as mentioned earlier, Granger Westberg's book *The Parish Nurse* and the chapters on faith and health in the book edited by Phyllis Ann Solari-Twadell and Mary Ann McDermott, entitled *Parish Nursing: Promoting Whole Person Health Within Faith Communities.*[2] You might also check with your particular denomination's leaders to see if they have health ministry promotional materials.

Some health cabinet members should be given the assignment to research the financial and programmatic logistics of starting such a ministry and to uncover the options for participating in existing parish nurse programs in their area. Most parish nurse programs will be glad to provide speakers on their programs and logistics, and many parish nurses serving other congregations will be glad to assist as well.

Having done its homework, the health cabinet will then want to meet with the pastor and church council (or whatever the church governing body is called) to present its findings and recommendations. It is extremely important to stay within a formal process for setting up a parish nurse ministry, for shortcutting steps and communication in the interest of saving time can hurt the effectiveness and sustainability of the program over time.

If the church council is amenable to further exploration, the health cabinet can then move forward to help the congregation explore the concept of parish nurse ministry. This can take place at a specially called congregational meeting, or at a series of adult education classes. The cabinet must be prepared to interpret to the congregation the connection between faith and health, and to help develop the congregation's particular call to health ministry in its unique place and time. Many congregations initially see little need for health ministry because of misunderstandings regarding the roles of the parish nurse. Often congregations are uncomfortable with engaging a nursing professional, questioning whether a church should be involved in the care of physical health, rather than leaving that realm to clinics and hospitals, which are primarily designed for physical care. This is where the homework done on theological underpinnings for the church's mandate to preach, teach, and heal are crucial.

If the congregation decides to pursue further study into a parish nurse program, discussions will need to continue. The congregation should consider whether it would prefer to have a parish nurse serve primarily as an internal resource, or whether it would like to see him or her do outreach to the community as well. Some parishioners may assume that a parish nurse would work only with people who do not have health insurance and may not understand how valuable a health ministry can be for all in the community. Others may assume that there will be a "clinic" set up in the fellowship hall, or that the parish nurse only will serve the elderly or another single segment of the membership or neighborhood. Conversations about the program must outline the roles of a parish nurse very clearly, to facilitate the decision about whether the ministry should primarily serve the congregation or be an outreach ministry, or a balance of both.

The congregation may need to vote on whether or not to start a program, especially if the recommendation is being made to pursue a paid parish nurse model. The leadership for such a presentation at a congregational meeting generally falls to the health cabinet. Here is a sample resolution for a congregation considering a parish nurse ministry:

> *Whereas* the call to the promotion of health and wholeness of body, mind, spirit, and community is a Christian call that responds to God's loving presence among us, and
>
> *Whereas* we follow in the footsteps of Jesus, our healer and teacher, who sent forth disciples to preach, teach, and heal, we hereby
>
> *Resolve* to explore congregational health ministry for a three-year trial period by calling a parish nurse to serve with us on a half-time basis in outreach to members of our church and the community beyond our walls.

2. Sharing the idea. The pastor and that person set up a meeting with people such as health professionals, social workers, teachers, or others they think might be interested in the idea.

3. Forming a health cabinet. Five to seven people, drawn from the group of interested people or others who are recommended by that group, are formed into a health cabinet.

4. Information gathering. The health cabinet meets to consider the theology of health ministry and to learn about parish nursing.

5. Information sharing. Findings of the initial period of study are shared with the pastor and the church governance body, such as a church council.

6. More information gathering. Questions identified in the meeting with the church council and pastor are researched.

7. Congregational meetings. Adult education classes and/or congregational meetings are held to explore the idea of beginning a parish nurse ministry.

8. Approval of program. The appropriate body, whether it is the church council or the congregation, takes a vote to start a parish nurse program and begin recruiting for the position.

9. Hiring. The health cabinet advertises for the position and, with the pastor, representatives of the health cabinet interview candidates. Upon review of the recommendation by the whole committee, a candidate is hired.

10. Strategic planning. The health cabinet works with the new parish nurse to assess the needs of the congregation and community and to plan and develop programs.

11. Performance review. Representatives of the health cabinet and the pastor review the performance of the parish nurse at six months, one year, and annually thereafter.

12. Program review. The health cabinet reviews congregational satisfaction with the parish nurse program after eighteen months and reviews program effectiveness about a year later.

Ongoing Roles of a Health Cabinet

While a health cabinet is critical for the start-up of an effective parish nurse program, it is also critical for its ongoing success. To recap, there are five areas where a health cabinet needs to provide direction and assistance to the health ministry of a congregation.

Theological reflection. The health cabinet should be willing to spend time reflecting on the biblical mandates to preach, teach, and heal, and to care for one's neighbor, both body and soul. The members of the health cabinet must be able to articulate the reasons for having parish nursing as part of a congregation's ministry.

Personnel. The health cabinet should recommend the type of parish nurse position to be offered (full-time, half-time) and compensation for a parish nurse (paid or unpaid, benefits, professional expenses). The health cabinet then would recruit and select the person to be a parish nurse, and participate in the review of her or his performance on an annual basis (as well as a six-month review during the first year).

Strategic planning. The health cabinet must be willing to meet with the parish nurse to help assess the health needs of a congregation and community and to help plan programmatic responses to those needs. This must be done at the start of the ministry and again on a periodic basis.

Volunteers. The health cabinet knows many more people in the congregation than a new parish nurse would and can help match gifts and talents of individual congregational members to needs within the health ministry. The health cabinet can serve as an invaluable resource to the new parish nurse in recruiting volunteers to be a part of the health ministry. These volunteers, in turn, may become future members of the health cabinet.

Fund-raising. A parish nurse program, whether a paid or an unpaid model, does have some costs associated with it. The health cabinet can help with fund-raising events, or provide direction in working with experts in grant writing, planned giving, or other fund-raising strategies.

Thus, the health cabinet is a critical and fundamental part of the parish nurse program. Being a member of a health cabinet requires a contribution of time and expertise. The impact that this committee can have on the life of a congregation and the surrounding community is tremendous, however. Satisfaction in seeing the congregation and community provide a vital and vibrant health ministry can provide a great return for the investment of time and energy.

Sent Out Two by Two
Sharing Ministry with a Parish Nurse

Pastor Bob: It was a bright and breezy Sunday afternoon when the initial meeting took place. She ran to the church parking lot wearing a "gi" (karate uniform) and barefoot. I thought, "This is the parish nurse?"

Parish Nurse Mary Ann: The look on his face told me that I was not what he expected. His wife and a member of the pastoral search committee were smiling. I remember he did not question my appearance. I sensed genuineness in his acceptance.

Pastor Bob: Near the end of our conversation she said, "Feel free to tell me to drop dead, go to hell, or leave the congregation." I replied, "You can tell me to drop dead, go to hell, but not to leave the congregation." This honest, sincere, and spirited exchange turned out to be the foundation of a vital shared ministry.

Jesus sent the disciples out two by two and they ministered to people's needs (Mark 6:7). There are joys and pitfalls in sharing ministry with another person, and so it is in the shared ministry of a pastor and a parish nurse.

As a team they minister to a parishioner holistically. Holistic ministry addresses a parishioner's body, mind, and spirit. The parish nurse brings knowledge of the medical discipline (body); the pastor brings to the team knowledge of theological discipline (mind); and it is the spirit that enables a dynamic interaction between the two. The parish nurse and pastor learn from each other for a sharpened awareness. As a team they walk alongside the parishioner in a process toward wholeness.

A parish nurse has nursing education that helps her understand a variety of diseases and conditions. A nurse's education and experience are invaluable to a congregation in assessing health conditions (not diagnosing!), intervening and advocating for needed services, seeking out appropriate referrals, and coordinating lay assistance when required. It is beneficial to the pastor and the parishioner to have a parish nurse who can help with serving the needs of the homebound, those in care facilities, the hospitalized, those in nursing homes, and others in crises involving health issues.

A pastor has theological education that helps him or her to provide a theological framework or interpretation for the concerns a parishioner might have. A pastor is also a valuable advocate and resource person. However, without a nursing or medical education, a pastor is hard pressed to make accurate health assessments or provide more than a cursory health education. Some pastors and parish nurses have specific instruction in spiritual assessment, as taught in a class such as Clinical Pastoral Education.

Both a parish nurse and a pastor perform their ministries with hearts open to the concerns of the parishioner. Their respective educational backgrounds and unique experiences work together for the good of the entire congregation.

It is extremely important to note that a parish nurse is not a pastor, nor is a pastor a parish nurse. Although there is certainly overlap in their ministries, each has a defined role and there is no need for competition. With personal confidence, each has a mutual respect of and trust in the other, leading to a team approach for ministering both outside (outreach) and within ("inreach") a congregation.

Turf issues, which occur when there is a sense of competition between the pastor and parish nurse, can be avoided. For example: A parishioner shared with Parish Nurse Mary Ann a pending medical procedure. After the nursing process was initiated, Mary Ann requested permission to share this information with Pastor Bob. She said, "We work as a team." Permission was granted, and they developed a holistic care plan. Following the plan, Mary Ann consulted with the parishioner before the procedure. Bob called the parishioner after the procedure. The parishioner shared the medical results, her fears, her joys, and her appreciation for their concern. Later, Pastor Bob relayed this information to Parish Nurse Mary Ann.

This comprehensive team approach of the pastor/parish nurse ministry avoids competition and is led by the Spirit for the benefit of the parishioner.

The personal preference of a parishioner to relate more closely to either the parish nurse or the pastor may lead to tension between the team. The preference occurs because of different personalities, styles of ministry, and factors related to male/female characteristics (where the genders of the pastor and parish nurse differ). The tension in ministry is real and must be recognized. Consequently, it is important that the parish nurse and the pastor stay in communication with each other. Making sure that the channels of communication stay open, honest, and clear about roles and responsibilities can ease tension. Good communication can be accomplished in a number of ways.

First of all, the offices of the pastor and parish nurse should be in close proximity, for one is not to overlook the "water cooler effect" in facilitating communication. A parish nurse whose office is in a far corner of the church building is physically less accessible, and there is the potential for weakening the shared ministry.

Second, the parish nurse and pastor must meet regularly to discuss parishioners' assessed needs, the mutually agreed upon interventions, and the evaluation of outcomes. Without regular communication, many important pieces of information may fall through the cracks, making it more difficult for either the pastor or the parish nurse to minister most effectively.

Third, it is important to define and then adhere to the lines of responsibility between the pastor and the parish nurse. Doing so avoids confusing parishioners and/or church staff. Well-defined roles lend strength to the team and clarity for the staff and the congregation.

Finally, an active and engaged health committee should help facilitate good communication through regular discussions of issues facing the parish nurse. Issues to be discussed could include the broad health concerns facing the congregation, planning future goals for health ministry, and support for the ministerial team relationship.

The congregation has a great need for both a pastor and a parish nurse. Together, they can make a great team or they can become adversaries. Both of these can and do happen. Therefore, care should be taken, using the collective wisdom of the pastor, the parish nurse, and the health committee, to confront negative issues quickly, before they become insurmountable obstacles to a healthy working relationship. Shared ministry does not just happen. It requires constant and intentional attention. The joy experienced by the pastor, the parish nurse, and the parishioners is worth all the effort.

Ministry in the Manner of Peter

The Paid Parish Nurse

THE APOSTLES IN THE EARLY Christian Church, such as Peter, were told to take no money with them, but to accept provisions from those to whom they ministered. It is one of the tenets underlying the practice of providing a salary for ordained clergy. Many factors argue for the paid parish nurse program within a congregation. I would like to note some of them here.

A professional health ministry. Paying a parish nurse underscores the message that parish nursing is a professional ministry of the church, requiring professional education and experience, in a manner similar to the requirements for ordained pastoral ministry. Just as the pastor is paid for his or her professional ministry, the parish nurse should be paid for his or her professional ministry. The parish nurse should also be installed or affirmed in ministry. (See appendix C for a sample service of installation.)

Expectations and supervision. A paid parish nurse can be supervised as an employee of the church and held to a standard parish nurse job description as a term of employment. Part of that job description should include the expectation that the parish nurse will participate in regular staff meetings, which greatly foster communication and teamwork.

In addition, remaining within the scope and standards of the practice of parish nursing reduces the liability exposure of both the parish nurse and the congregation. The scope and standards for parish nursing were published by the Health Ministries Association and the American Nurses Association, and should be required reading for the parish nurse, pastor, and health committee.[1]

Increased time commitment. A paid parish nurse may have fewer outside distractions from her work at the church than a volunteer, because the congregational setting is where she is receiving her income (or half her income, if she also is working at another part-time job). The parish nurse is not forced to spend a great deal of her energies earning full-time income elsewhere. She or he can be required to work a certain number of hours, including specific times, whereas a volunteer may not feel the same obligation to work those hours.

Confidentiality. Congregational members may be more willing to share concerns with a nurse who is not a member of their congregation and who is perceived as a professional member of the ministerial team. A paid parish nurse may be perceived as more professional than a volunteer, since a paid parish nurse is generally present only in that role, whereas the volunteer who is probably a member of that congregation would be wearing two hats—church member and parish nurse. However, this could be potentially as much of an issue for the paid parish nurse who is serving her home congregation.

Larger pool of applicants. Generally, to attract someone from outside the congregation, the position must be paid. If the health cabinet would like to be able to select a parish nurse from a number of candidates, they should certainly plan on the paid model for parish nursing.

Increased visibility. Whenever a financial investment is involved in implementing a ministry within a congregation, there generally is a need for more people to be involved in the decision making than would be the case for a volunteer program. That process automatically increases the visibility of the parish nurse ministry within church leadership circles from the start of exploratory conversations. Including the parish nurse ministry in the congregation's budget means that the program must have support from a wide number of people before it can be approved. It also ensures that there are many people on board when the ministry actually begins within a congregation. In addition, needing to budget for the program keeps parish nursing before the congregation on a regular (at least annual) basis, when the budget is reviewed.

The paid model for parish nursing, at least half-time, if not full-time, is one that works very well. It allows the congregation to choose from among a pool of qualified applicants from the wider community. It recognizes the parish nurse as a professional in the health ministry of the congregation, and encourages congregational members to relate to that person in confidence.

If a congregation opts for a half-time paid position for a parish nurse, that arrangement allows the parish nurse with other interests to pursue them while still maintaining a strong commitment to health ministry. This model also allows sufficient time for visibility and sustainability of the parish nurse program.

Many churches do not feel that they can support a paid model, however, and have implemented an unpaid parish nurse model, which also can be effective under the right conditions. The chapter that follows will explore some of those conditions.

Ministry in the Manner of Paul
The Unpaid Parish Nurse

THE APOSTLE PAUL MAINTAINED HIS tent-making work to support himself financially in his outreach ministry, establishing a strong precedent for the unpaid model in ministry. Certainly any program that raises the visibility of health ministry is worthwhile, even if the person spearheading the effort has only a few hours per week to commit to the effort.

While it is my belief that a paid model for parish nursing is optimal for the reasons explored in the preceding chapter, there are a number of factors that can argue for an unpaid parish nurse program within a congregation. I would like to discuss some of them here.

Priesthood of all believers. All members of the church are called to be ministers. An unpaid parish nurse model affirms the priesthood of all believers, in that each member of the congregation is called to a particular ministry within the church. Whereas not all the members of the congregation are remunerated for their ministries, neither would a volunteer parish nurse be remunerated.

Installation and recognition. A volunteer parish nurse can be affirmed and installed into her ministry just as other lay leaders, such as teachers in a Christian education ministry, would be affirmed and installed into their respective ministries within the church. (See appendix C for a sample service of affirmation and installation.)

Ease of program start-up. It is far easier to start a parish nurse program when you have a volunteer than when a line item needs to be added to the budget. Fewer people need to be involved in deciding to start an unpaid program than when a financial commitment is involved, so a program can easily begin, especially on a trial basis, when the parish nurse is willing to work under this model.

One potential problem, however, is that a congregation may be unwilling to pay later for services they first receive at no cost, especially when they were not involved in coming to the decision to try the program. Another risk that needs to be considered is that the entire health ministry runs a higher chance of ending when the volunteer leaves than it does if there is a paid parish nurse position into which someone else would be expected to be hired.

Commitment to the program. Generally, a parish nurse is someone who sincerely believes in the integration of faith and health and genuinely wants to make a contribution to the well-being of the congregation and wider community.

However, this is also true for the paid parish nurse, and commitment by the volunteer parish nurse often is not as strong as if that person were being paid to do health ministry. This is true for a number of reasons, often including the need to earn a living, and time demands of other family and volunteer activities.

Established presence in the church. An unpaid parish nurse is generally a member of the congregation, and may be well known by other members. This parish nurse may already be intimately familiar with many of the health concerns of the congregation and would have a head start on an employed parish nurse from outside the congregation, who would need more time to become familiar with the health status of the congregation.

It might be difficult, however, for other congregational members to share concerns with a parish nurse who belongs to the same congregation, because that person may not be seen as a neutral professional. A parish nurse who belongs to a congregation must be doubly aware of the professional and ethical boundaries of working in such a position.

Another consideration for the pastor and health cabinet is that it is very difficult to terminate a volunteer, and it is especially painful to do so when the volunteer is a congregational member. Therefore, each parish nurse should agree to a standard parish nurse job description and agree to regular reviews by the pastor and a member of the health cabinet, a necessary component of health ministry regardless of whether the parish nurse is paid or unpaid.

In addition, a parish nurse who is working on a volunteer basis may work fewer hours than a paid parish nurse and may feel free to leave for an extended vacation at any time. The unpaid parish nurse should be encouraged to consider such absences carefully if the health ministry is to project a professional image. All vacations should be discussed in advance, and wherever possible, arrangements should be made with another parish nurse to provide assistance if needed by the pastor or other congregational members in order to maintain the visibility and credibility of the program. (If another parish nurse is not available in the area, arrangements should be made with another R.N. or with a trained member of the health cabinet to provide assistance during the parish nurse's absences.)

Lower cost to the congregation. Obviously, the unpaid model is much less expensive, since the congregation is providing neither a salary nor benefits, although the congregation is urged to provide funds for a parish nurse basic preparation class and continuing education.

The parish nurse should be expected to work within the scope and standards of parish nurse practice, to avoid putting his or her nursing license and the congregation at exposure for a liability claim. Finally, the congregation should require any parish nurse to carry professional liability insurance, and the church should purchase coverage as well.[1]

The congregation should note that while they are investing fewer dollars than they would if they were paying a salary to a parish nurse, they should still invest in support of and affirmation for the parish nurse ministry. Because the unpaid ministry tends to be less visible, it may be more difficult to find affirmation and it is also more difficult to find other parish nurses who have time to meet. Given the other pressures on an individual's time, this may lead to a higher turnover under the volunteer model, and the congregation should do all within its power to affirm and support its parish nurse.

More than 65 percent of the current parish nurses in the United States are doing health ministry on an unpaid basis. Some volunteer parish nurses are working in other paid health-care positions, some are retired from other paid health-care positions, while others are at home with small children, taking a hiatus from paid employment. There are some parish nurse programs, such as St. Joseph Health System in Atlanta, that allow congregations that are interested in the unpaid parish nurse model to contract with the program for supervision, continuing education, and liability insurance coverage, in exchange for a modest annual fee. If your congregation is exploring the volunteer model, you may wish to consider this approach and investigate options for support in your area.

There are many different arrangements for engaging a parish nurse and shaping a health ministry. One of those arrangements will be right for your congregation.

How Much Does It Cost?

Summary of the Costs of a Parish Nurse Program

THE COST OF A PARISH nurse program can vary widely, from a few dollars (for there always will be some costs), to over forty thousand dollars,[1] depending upon a number of factors: whether the parish nurse is paid or unpaid, whether benefits are provided, whether the parish nurse works full-time or part-time (and the number of part-time hours can vary), and whether another organization is sharing the cost. The following text lists some of the basic considerations.

Office space. At a minimum, a parish nurse will need a desk, a telephone with a line on which an answering machine or voice mail service can record confidential messages, and a locking file cabinet for records. Optimally, this would be in a separate office, where he or she could meet privately with others. In addition, a computer with e-mail and Internet access is extremely helpful. The cost can be up to $1500 (depending upon whether new office furniture and equipment, including computer and printer, are purchased), plus overhead for office space, utilities, and maintenance, as well as the cost of office supplies, postage, and telephone calls. The suggested budgeted amount for office expenses (not including salary, benefits, or continuing education) is $2000–$3000 for the first year and $500–$1000 each following year. (Of course you will want to adjust for inflation in future years.)

Parish nurse basic preparation. Parish nursing is not generally taught as part of the R.N. or B.S.N. curriculum. Therefore, a curriculum was developed by the International Parish Nurse Resource Center with the help of other faculty and experts in the field of parish nursing. Authors were drawn from over twenty parish nurse programs, colleges, and universities around the country. The curriculum addressed the need for standardization in introducing the field of parish nursing to those interested in embarking in the area of health ministry. Classes using this curriculum, highly recommended for all beginning parish nurses to equip them for their work, are currently available at more than eighty colleges, universities, and parish nurse programs around the country and abroad. Some are taught as a one-week session, while others have a weekend or evening format, and some are considering an on-line format. Costs range from about $475 to over $1300, depending upon the program and area, and depending upon whether the parish nurse wishes to receive college credit. This is a one-time expense. For more information on offerings, visit a listing of current classes at <www.parishnurses.org>.

Salary. Currently, in the Midwest, a parish nurse will earn fourteen to fifteen dollars per hour. This is about three dollars per hour less than a starting hospital nurse would earn in the region. Parish nurses in other parts of the country may earn significantly more, depending on the funding source. However, parish nurses approach their work as a ministry and a calling, and while they would welcome a salary equivalent to one found on a scale paid by a hospital, many registered nurses are willing to accept a lower salary from a church. In addition, parish nurses perform physically easier work and often less stressful work than nurses working in a hospital, so that even though most parish nurses come to the position with significant experience, many will consider this lower salary. An important factor in setting salary is that we have found no church willing to pay its parish nurse (or anyone else on staff) more than its pastor is paid.

Deaconess Parish Nurse Ministries (DPNM), the organization with which the International Parish Nurse Resource Center is affiliated, currently employs nearly thirty parish nurses, providing salary support over several years to each congregation in the form of a declining grant. That is, DPNM currently provides two-thirds of the parish nurse's salary during the first year, one third in the second year, and continues paying the cost of her or his benefits in the third year and following years. DPNM has had the policy of paying each of our new parish nurses the same starting salary, regardless of the size of the church. Therefore, a half-time parish nurse at $14.50 per hour will earn $15,080 per year. The congregation will need to budget for salary increases to offset the cost of inflation. A congregation, of course, can set its own salary level if hiring a parish nurse independently of a parish nurse program.

Salary sharing. Salary can be shared with another congregation, but we do not recommend that a parish nurse serve more than two congregations at once. We feel it is important to ask a parish nurse to be present at worship at least twice a month to get well acquainted with the congregation. In addition, it does not seem practical to expect a parish nurse program to flourish by investing fewer than ten hours per week per congregation, which may be the case when a nurse is stretched between too many congregations. These are issues, however, that each congregation will need to decide for themselves.

Benefits. Please see chapter 11 on benefits for a more complete discussion of this issue. We would add that if a church is paying a parish nurse independently (not as part of a parish nurse program at another organization), the church is responsible for paying for the parish nurse's Worker's Compensation and Social Security (FICA), just as they would be for any other employee. We would encourage including the parish nurse in the same benefits plans as the ordained clergy are receiving, such as health insurance and pension plans. Most denominational plans will include parish nurses—please contact them for specific plan details.

Continuing education. An important factor for success as the sole health professional employed by a congregation is to stay current in one's field. The church should budget a certain amount of money each year for the parish nurse to update skills. The amount could include funds for the purchase of books, subscriptions to nursing journals, and attendance at classes at local hospitals. We also encourage parish nurses to attend the annual Westberg Symposium, where a wide variety of speakers discuss parish nursing and the latest books and materials on parish nursing are available for review. Another excellent resource for continuing education is the annual conference sponsored by the Health Ministries Association. Recommended budget for continuing education: $700–800.

As you can see, there is a wide range of costs related to parish nursing, and there is no "one-size-fits-all" approach. If you find a partner with whom you can share costs, such as benefits or continuing education, you are already ahead of the game. Local charitable foundations may be a source of help, especially at the onset of the program. Some examples of foundations that have helped to support the start-up of parish nurse programs include the Wellborn Foundation in Evansville, Indiana, the Flower Foundation in Toledo, Ohio, and the Lutheran Foundation in St. Louis, Missouri, as well as the Deaconess Foundation in St. Louis, Missouri, as previously mentioned.

If a congregation chooses a half-time paid model for parish nursing, using the current salary standards for the Midwest, the first-year costs would be approximately $18,000 to $30,000, depending on salary and whether or not benefits were paid by the church. Of course, this cost may be shared with another congregation, and/or a partner may be found to help with salary and benefits. The office expenses would be reduced in successive years, but the church would need to budget for cost-of-living salary increases.

If a congregation decides to go with the unpaid model for parish nursing, funds will still be necessary for office expenses and education, both basic preparation and continuing education.

We highly recommend the parish nurse basic preparation class, even for a volunteer parish nurse, so she or he is able to learn the scope of practice and understand the job description and possibilities for health ministry in relation to peers. Without this educational preparation and ongoing networking and support, a volunteer parish nurse is unlikely to be able to offer a well-rounded parish nurse ministry and may expose the congregation to liability by operating outside the scope of parish nurse practice. Costs for an unpaid parish nurse ministry during the start-up year would be approximately $3000–4000, depending on the cost of the basic preparation class and any continuing education.

Can the Church Afford It?

Financing a Parish Nurse Program

O NE OF THE MOST DAUNTING obstacles to beginning any parish nurse program is how to pay for it, especially when there are so many competing demands on the congregational budget. Various options for funding a paid parish nurse program in a congregation are included here, and the list of models that exist for funding such a ministry is constantly growing.

Partnership with a Health-care Organization

The first option that should be explored for funding a parish nurse program is through a partnership with another organization. In a metropolitan area, there may be hospitals or health systems that are interested in expanding their parish nurse departments. Churches should contact the spiritual care or community education departments of hospitals in their area to see if such programs exist. Usually hospitals will provide no more than a half-time parish nurse to your congregation and may require that at least one other (if not more) church share the parish nurse. Churches should be aware that having a parish nurse for less than ten hours a week will probably provide few benefits to the congregation, and should consider other avenues for funding if asked to share a parish nurse with more than one other congregation. As stated earlier, we have found the optimal amount of time for a parish nurse to be employed by a congregation to be at least twenty hours per week, with at least two Sundays per month in attendance at worship services.

Most interested health-care organizations provide some form of assistance for salary and/or benefits for an initial period, usually two to five years, in order to help a church set up a program. The hospital may also provide liability insurance for the parish nurse and congregation. Please see chapter 11 on benefits for parish nurses for more information on this topic.

Foundation Funding

When funding through a health-care organization is not available, there may be a foundation willing to help start a program. It generally cannot be expected that a foundation will continue payment beyond the first few years, however. Most philanthropic organizations will assist with start-up only, not with ongoing salary and other operational expenses.

For more information on locating foundations in your area, you might want to visit the Foundation Center's Web site at <www.fdncenter.org>, or contact your local Regional Association of Grantmaking. Many states of the country are represented by Regional Associations of Grantmakers, which are membership organizations of community, private, and family foundations and corporate donors, who choose to voluntarily participate in strengthening philanthropy. Often these associations are a wealth of information about foundations and other donors in the area in which you live.

It is important to note that these associations are membership organizations of funders, not direct funders themselves. They may be a helpful source of information to you about donors, but they will not provide funding, nor should you request it from them. A number of these associations, however, do have programs for organizations who are seeking funding, such as forums for the introduction of new foundations into the community, or access to libraries with databases and information on where and how to apply for grants. They may also offer programs on the fundamentals of fund-raising.[1] Often these programs do have a fee, but they are generally very helpful.

You may wish to contact the Forum of Regional Associations of Grantmakers at <www.rag.org> to locate member associations in your state or to inquire about other philanthropic roundtables or collaborative ventures in your area.

In addition, a number of directories exist that list local and national foundations, and these generally can be found in your local public library.

Congregational Donors

A health cabinet may be able to identify some congregational members, perhaps even just one financially secure member of the congregation, who would be willing to support the cost of this ministry. Often individuals who have benefited from the parish nurse ministry will be willing to make a pledge toward underwriting the program.

A second option for congregational donors is setting up a subscription for the parish nurse ministry. This would involve spreading the cost over a number of parishioners, each buying a "share" in the cost of the parish nurse ministry, which they would pay on a weekly, monthly, or annual basis.

A third option is to consider using income from predonated funds, that is, from a congregation's endowment funds, if they are not already committed to other areas of ministry. Starting an endowment for parish nurse ministry is a good way to ensure sustainability.

Memorials and Tributes

Churches often find that many memorials for deceased congregational members may be designated for the parish nurse program. A gift to the parish nurse ministry is also a wonderful way to honor someone, and often gifts are given as a tribute to the parish nurse. Memorials and tributes can be given to program operating expenses, or to an endowment for parish nursing.

Planned Giving

The greatest potential for the sustainability of the parish nurse program is through planned giving to an endowment. Individuals whose lives have been changed by this ministry are often looking to find a way to keep that ministry alive for others. The health committee would be wise to identify people who may have a particular interest in the future support of this ministry, just as any pastor would speak with church members about planned giving for support of the congregation.

For more information about planned giving, talk with denominational leadership in your area. Many denominational offices have individuals identified with experience in this area and are willing to assist congregations. You may also have development professionals, accountants, or lawyers in your congregations who are willing to assist. Finally, the local library will have printed resources on planned giving. You will want all individuals considering making such a gift to speak with their own tax advisor or attorney for the options most beneficial to their particular financial situation.

Fund-Raising

Many congregations fund their parish nurse program primarily through fund-raising events. Some churches find they are able to fund the entire program with one fund-raising event per year, while others raise the amount over the course of the year with regular fund-raisers. Here are ten fund-raising ideas to help you get started:

"Benefit Your Health" dinner. Most benefit dinners consist of delicious fatty, salty, sugar-filled food. Have the parish nurse work with the cooks in your congregation or a local caterer to plan an attractive, tasty, heart-healthy meal as a fund-raiser.

Cookbooks for health. Many church cookbooks are filled with pages of various condensed soup and noodle casseroles. Here is an opportunity to include parishioners in digging out and sharing their favorite healthy recipes.

Silent auction—healthy style. Silent auctions can be very successful as a fund-raiser and can help to spread the word about the parish nurse program as volunteers seek donors. A special emphasis might be placed on securing health-related items such as baskets of teas, gift certificates or coupons for health-food stores, exercise clubs, visits to massage therapists, or health spas, or other items that promote wellness. Don't forget that a healthy person is also a member of a healthy community, so include items for community building, such as tickets to baseball games and gift certificates for restaurant dinners.

Health trivia nights. A trivia night with a focus on questions about wellness and spirituality could serve both as a fund-raiser and an educational event. See the suggestions above for prize items.

The Mile-and-a-half "I Hate to Walk-a-thon." How about using a very short walk-a-thon (any odd distance would do) to reach those who might otherwise never participate in such an event, but who would be able to walk a relatively short distance? Pledges could be made in increments of one tenth of a mile. Resting spots could be set up along the way, with music or other entertainment there. Churches in near proximity to one another could form the start and end for such an event, with juice and fruit at the start and a healthy brunch (donations accepted, of course) at the end.

A fund-raising walk-a-thon can have health benefits, especially when the parish nurse implements a "training" program for those interested in walking before the event. Who knows, perhaps the "I Hate to Walk-A-Thon" will spur a regular walking group!

First aid kits. The parish nurse could help volunteers working with the health cabinet to assemble first-aid kits with items purchased in bulk. These first-aid kits would then be made available for sale to the congregation and neighbors at a reasonable profit as a community service and a fund-raiser for the parish nurse program.

Sale of other health-related items. Some Internet sites, such as <www.fundraising-ideas.org>, include many fund-raising products offered for sale at various companies. You might find items that would be of interest to your congregation or community that could become a regular fund-raiser. Most of the companies on this site have catalogs available on-line or through their toll-free numbers. Be sure to evaluate the initial investment versus the expected profit, and consider shipping costs. Many companies pay shipping costs on fund-raising items, but their products may cost more to the organization. You probably would want to find a product that had some relationship to health in order to provide a service to the community as part of the fund-raiser, such as a "Kid Safe Fingerprint-a-Thon." (See their Web site at <www.thekidsafenetwork.com>.)

House concerts. Community building, as mentioned earlier, is an extremely important tool for building a healthy congregation and community. House concerts, often held in conjunction with a potluck meal, are a great way to meet and have fellowship with others, and to raise funds for parish nursing at the same time.

Complete ideas for how to sponsor a house concert are found on Web sites such as <http://houseconcerts.org>, which offers an online "House Concert Guide." One very important caveat—make sure you turn off the ringer on your phone!

Breakfasts. One couple living in Vancouver, British Columbia, was able to raise over sixteen thousand dollars for Parkinson's research by inviting friends and colleagues to a breakfast, which they called "Porridge for Parkinson's." Marg Meikle, who has Parkinson's, and her husband Noel MacDonald, invited two hundred people to their home, planned for 150, and 180 came. Many others sent contributions. They served oatmeal (pottage), fruit compote, juice, coffee, and tea and raised funds and awareness. Their costs for the event were only three hundred dollars. For more information on hosting an event of this type, visit their Web site at <www.porridgeforparkinsons.com>.

Special products. You might find an artist or a manufacturer in your congregation who will be willing to work with you to develop a symbolic product that you could sell to promote parish nursing. For examples, many housing organizations have sold handmade lapel pins made by an artist who distributes her pins solely through such organizations. Lydia's House, a transitional housing program for women leaving situations of domestic abuse, was able to sell enough pins in four years to purchase another housing facility. Carol Ann Cole, a breast cancer survivor in Canada, raised over one million dollars for the Canadian Cancer Society by selling small pewter pendants in the shape of actual hearts, which she called "Comfort Hearts." Finding a symbol related to your work and selling it as broadly as possible is one key to this type of fund-raising.

Successful fund-raisers depend, in great measure, on three factors: First, offer an innovative product or event. People are tired of attending the same fund-raising dinner every year or buying the same kind of wrapping paper. If you do the same thing, put a spin on it. One small rural church in Josephberg, Alberta has an annual chicken dinner, but they publicize it throughout the region, saying they are trying to set the world's record for the most people fed at a single church chicken dinner—last year the event drew over 2,700 people.

Second, have good volunteers to put together the fund-raiser and get the word out. Carole Ann Cole's campaign to sell "Comfort Hearts" was aided by good publicity in the media, and seeking publicity is where a lot of people helped.

Third, have a very visible parish nurse program. People are more likely to support a cause they know something about and to which they can relate. Here is where the parish nurse and health committee really need to do their homework, year-round.

Phase-In of the Parish Nurse Program

One option that has worked for some congregations has been to start a parish nurse ministry with a few hours a week and gradually increase paid hours as visibility of the program and base of support grows. Some churches have started parish nurse programs with five hours per week and have added as little as an hour at a time, as funding allows.

At $14.50 an hour, which is the current starting rate for parish nurses in our area,[2] a parish nurse working five hours a week involves a starting financial commitment of $3,770 per year from the congregation (not including the cost for benefits, if any, basic preparation, continuing education, and office expenses. See chapter 9 on the costs of a parish nurse program.

While such limited time is not optimal, starting with a few hours per week gives the pastor someone with whom he or she can consult. The parish nurse can also offer services during that time, such as blood pressure screenings, newsletter articles, and a few educational offerings.

"Free Trial Offer"

Finally, some parish nurses have offered their services to congregations on an unpaid trial basis for a limited time, with the understanding that at the end of that time the health committee would evaluate to see if the church should consider continuing on a paid basis. One risk of this approach is that the answer might at that time be "no." In the worst case scenario, the nurse has made a voluntary contribution to the support of the church, but more often than not, the congregation has seen by then the importance of financially supporting such a ministry in their midst.

It must be noted, however, that a congregation is often reluctant to pay for something it has been receiving for free, and a great deal of education will be necessary over the course of the year to make the case for a paid parish nurse ministry there.

As you can see, the options for funding a paid parish nurse ministry are limited only by the imagination of those seeking the funding. Some congregations are fortunate enough to have members with financial resources to fund the program, others use endowment funds, and others raise the funds. Congregations should not dismiss the paid professional model for parish nursing before considering a number of fund-raising options. In addition, most health cabinets are generally willing to share their experience and expertise in financing the costs of the ministry.

An excellent resource that provides further information on fund-raising is the book, *Starting a Nonprofit at Your Church* by Joy Skjegstad. Skjegstad's chapter on fund-raising contains tips on requesting funds from individual donors to foundations, including elements of writing a grant proposal. The bibliography also includes a number of other helpful resources.[3]

From the paid model through a health-care organization to a model using a patchwork quilt of spirited fund-raising, many opportunities exist for developing a parish nurse ministry in your congregation.

Can the Parish Nurse Afford It?

Providing Benefits for a Parish Nurse

A CHURCH THAT IS PAYING a parish nurse, whether on a part-time or full-time basis, probably will want to also consider providing benefits as well. The following brief description will outline a few of the issues involved.

It is important to note here that the following is only an introduction to areas that should be explored when considering providing benefits for a parish nurse. This is not meant to be professional advice to a congregation on any particular federal or state laws or a recommendation on any particular insurance plan.

Benefits Provided by Another Organization

First of all, a congregation should compare the benefits packages of various programs that sponsor parish nurses, if you have the luxury of being located in a geographic location where choices are an option. These programs may provide benefits or can identify options for such items as health insurance, life insurance, professional liability insurance, retirement savings, short- and long-term disability insurance, long-term care insurance, continuing education, and tuition reimbursement. Many parish nurse programs offer some, if not all, of these benefits or may make them available for the church to purchase at a reduced rate. The sponsoring organization administers the benefits and saves the church from the headache of negotiating them.

When a parish nurse program at a hospital or network provides these benefits, the parish nurse usually must be an employee of the organization, not of the church. If the church pays a portion (or all) of the salary, and even a portion (or all) of the benefits for the parish nurse, the arrangement usually requires a reimbursement to the program that actually employs the parish nurse, in order to qualify for group employee benefits. Otherwise, the cost of providing benefits to individuals might be much more expensive.

Health Insurance

Benefits packages for parish nurses vary, but it may be difficult to employ a parish nurse without providing health insurance, unless she has already has such insurance through another source. Nurses today are all too familiar with the problems faced by the uninsured. The cost of health insurance, however, as everyone in the United States is aware, is very high and still rising. A congregation is encouraged to look at various options for providing health insurance by speaking with an insurance broker or independent advisor.

Retirement Savings Plan

The congregation may wish to participate in a retirement savings plan for the parish nurse. This is especially important if the parish nurse is not employed elsewhere as well. Many retirement savings plans exist, including denominational plans and private plans. The health committee would be well advised to contact a professional with expertise in retirement planning for options to consider.

Worker Classification

The health cabinet must determine whether the parish nurse is an independent contractor, for whom an IRS Form 1099 is required, or an employee, for whom a W-2 is required. An independent contractor would pay for her or his own social security taxes, worker's compensation insurance, and other benefits.

In addition, parish nurses, like pastors, should be designated as "exempt" employees with regard to federal and state wage and hour laws. Under this designation, "exempt" employees are excluded from specific provisions of federal and state wage and hour laws. For example, overtime would not be paid to an "exempt" employee.

If the parish nurse is an employee of the church, then the church must pay the employer portion of social security (FICA, currently at 7.65 percent of annual salary), and worker's compensation insurance.

Please check with your denominational office for employer requirements to be certain that your congregation is in compliance in this area.

Professional Liability Insurance

Professional liability is often a perceived barrier to setting up a parish nurse program, but in actuality, if the parish nurse remains within the professional scope and standards for parish nursing practice, the risk of a lawsuit is minimal. Health education, advocacy resource referral, and coordination of volunteers are not areas that would expose a parish nurse and the congregation to great risk—parish nurses encourage people to seek help, not defer it.

As of this printing, there have been very few lawsuits filed against parish nurses in the United States, the most litigious of countries in which parish nurses are currently operating. None of those lawsuits have been successful.

Professional liability insurance for a congregation who has a parish nurse, currently costing between two hundred and four hundred dollars annually, is highly recommended. Often, denominational insurance programs will offer liability coverage for parish nurses. Many parish nurses choose to carry their own professional liability insurance in addition to the coverage provided by the church, but the church should be a named insured on their policy as well. Some insurance carriers will ask for a sample parish nurse job description before providing coverage to a church or nurse, but this is easily provided.[1] Insurance protects not only against liability, but also defends the policy holder in the event of an adverse action or the contemplation of one. Many policies also provide risk management services.

If your congregation is partnering with a hospital or other parish nurse network, that organization's program will often provide professional liability insurance for its parish nurses. Be sure to ask about this.

Other Benefits

Vacation and sick leave. It is highly recommended that the church set aside at least two weeks annually for the parish nurse to have a vacation, and at least one week of sick time annually. This time may be increased as the tenure of the parish nurse increases.

Other insurance. Other types of insurance, especially disability and life insurance, but also dental insurance, vision insurance, and long-term care insurance may also be considered for the parish nurse. The church may opt to start with a few benefits and add others in future years.

Continuing Education and Support

Continuing education for parish nurses, like other professionals, is extremely important and valuable to continued growth and development of the ministry. Even if the church operates an independent parish nurse program and its parish nurse is not an employee of a parish nurse program, it is well worth checking into the local options for networking.

Continuing education for parish nurses is important for several reasons. Much of the information needed to stay current in the field is gained by attending update classes designed specifically for parish nurses. Learning about new resources with which to serve one's congregation is often done through networking, at which parish nurses quickly become expert. Finally, parish nurse ministry, like many other forms of ministry, can be very isolating over time.

The Westberg Parish Nurse Symposium, which takes place in the fall of each year, is a continuing education event open to parish nurses and others interested in health ministry. It is an important arena for presentation of the latest research and thought on parish nursing and for networking with parish nurses from around the United States and abroad.[2] Another arena for continuing education is the Health Ministries Association Conference, which takes place in the spring and is designed for health ministry in its broadest form, including clergy, chaplains, and lay health workers.[3]

Many networks of parish nurses are springing up around the United States and abroad. For example, in St. Louis, the Greater St. Louis Parish Nurse Network encompasses nearly one hundred parish nurses who are employed by several different programs in the region, as well as volunteer parish nurses. The group meets bimonthly and sponsors an annual retreat. Congregations should encourage the parish nurse to attend such meetings. While this is not an item for which a congregation needs to budget additional funds beyond modest annual dues, the time on the job spent by the parish nurse in such networking and renewal is time well spent for the congregation as well.

Setting aside funds for continuing education for the parish nurse should be an important part of the church's budget. Even churches that have a volunteer parish nurse should consider designating some funds for continuing education, because this may be a helpful way to honor and support the work of a volunteer parish nurse. We recommend that between seven hundred and one thousand dollars per year be set aside for continuing education.

Congregations also may want to consider setting up a book budget for parish nurses to purchase resources. Some parish nurse programs also have offered tuition reimbursement to help parish nurses complete further degrees in nursing, to study clinical pastoral education, or to take seminary classes.

Providing benefits for a parish nurse provides a measure of financial security, and continuing education helps her or him to become better equipped to minister with the congregation. Both of these elements greatly strengthen the parish nurse program in a congregation.

12

How to Grow a Parish Nurse
Parish Nurse Basic Preparation

A NY CONGREGATION WANTING to have a health ministry is urged to hire a parish nurse who has gone through a parish nurse basic preparation class or who is willing to do so upon beginning employment. A parish nurse must be a Registered Nurse, with a Bachelor of Science in Nursing the preferred qualification, and at least two years' experience in a health-care setting is recommended.

Parish nursing is not generally a class taught in colleges of nursing at this time (although this is changing rapidly). Therefore, it is necessary for a nurse to have further education in the field of parish nursing before embarking on the practice of health ministry.

Parish nurse basic preparation classes are taught in many locations around the country. The curriculum, developed by the International Parish Nurse Resource Center in consultation with the National League for Nursing (NLN) and the American Nurses Association (ANA), is a comprehensive set of lesson plans written by two dozen experienced parish nurse educators from institutions around the United States and abroad. The curriculum is taught by Educational Partners of the International Parish Nurse Resource Center. Educational Partners are those academic and health-care institutions that use the curriculum developed by the International Parish Nurse Resource Center as described above for the parish nurse basic preparation class. Some of the classes are offered over the course of one week, some are over two or more weekends, and some are evening classes meeting once a week for several weeks or months. You should be able to find a class that will work with your schedule.[1]

There are also academic and health-care institutions that offer parish nursing classes using curriculum developed by their own institutions. A strong parish nurse basic preparation class should cover a broad range of the issues. Here is a summary of the curriculum developed by the International Parish Nurse Resource Center, to help a congregation and parish nurse know what types of information a basic class should offer.

The primary objectives of this curriculum are five-fold:

1. Understanding of the integration of faith and health as central to the parish nurse role

2. Knowledge and skills needed to practice as a beginning parish nurse

3. Intercollegial peer support

4. Identification of networks for continuing development and support

5. Commitment to continued spiritual growth to support the role of parish nurse within a congregation.

The parish nurse basic preparation class addresses the following topics as part of the standard curriculum:

Module 1.   The Role of the Congregation in Health, Healing, and Wholeness

Module 2.   Theology of Health, Healing, and Wholeness

Module 3.   History and Philosophy of Parish Nursing

Module 4.   Ethics in Parish Nursing

Module 5.   Self-Care for Parish Nurses

Module 6.   Assessment: Individual, Family, Congregation

Module 7.   Accountability and Documentation

Module 8.   Function of the Parish Nurse: Integrator of Faith and Health

Module 9.   Function of the Parish Nurse: Personal Health Counselor

Module 10. Function of the Parish Nurse: Health Educator

Module 11. Function of the Parish Nurse: Referral Agent

Module 12. Function of the Parish Nurse: Coordinator of Volunteers

Module 13. Function of the Parish Nurse: Developer of Support Groups

Module 14. Function of the Parish Nurse: Health Advocate

Module 15. Getting Started

Module 16. Functioning within a Ministerial Team

Module 17. Health Promotion and Maintenance

Module 18. Prayer and Worship Leadership

Module 19. Legal Considerations for Parish Nurses

Module 20. Grant Writing for Parish Nursing

Module 21. Grief and Loss

All the institutions offering this curriculum have arranged for continuing education hours in the states where the institutions are located. In addition, the Educational Partners offering this curriculum also make available academic credit for this class (usually for an additional per credit hour fee). Faculty for the basic preparation classes taught by Educational Partners all must hold at least a master's degree in nursing and have completed a Faculty Preparation class with educators from other academic institutions or health-care organizations.

The cost of the parish nurse basic preparation class varies from place to place, depending upon local expenses for speakers and facilities. You may wish to contact more than one program to inquire about the cost. Generally, the registration fee includes all materials and meals during the class hours. Most programs also have college or retreat-type housing available for an additional fee. At the time of this writing, basic preparation class fees ranged from approximately five hundred to more than thirteen hundred dollars (higher if academic credit is earned).

Generally, class sizes are kept small to make possible a high level of class participation. Since that is the case, basic preparation classes often fill quickly, and early registration is advised whenever possible.

13

Now What?

Helping a New Parish Nurse Get Started

One of the pioneers in parish nursing is Alvyne Rethemeyer, who began working with parish nurses at Deaconess Health System shortly after the program was initiated. For a number of years she coordinated the Deaconess Parish Nurse Ministry Network, growing the ministry from eight nurses to nearly thirty. Alvyne taught the parish nurse basic preparation class in St. Louis and around the Midwest and was one of the original contributing authors to the parish nurse basic preparation curriculum. Currently, Alvyne has moved to another area within Deaconess Parish Nurse Ministries, LLC, serving as director of the International Parish Nurse Resource Center, overseeing such activities as the Westberg Symposium and educational classes for parish nurses, coordinators, and faculty. This chapter was written by Alvyne, who has had many years of experience "launching" new parish nurses.

A PARISH NURSE WHO HAD just been hired to begin a parish nurse ministry once wrote, "I sat at my desk with an empty rolodex and wondered, 'Now what do I do?'" The first few weeks in any new position can be confusing and stressful, especially if this is a brand new ministry for the congregation as well. Most nurses want very much to do the ministry well and be an asset to the congregation. But if a nurse has always worked in a structured institutional environment, she is used to being given assignments and completing them. Deciding what needs to be done on a daily basis may be a new and scary experience.

Getting Ready

The congregation and clergy have a definite role in this transition from employee to health minister. First, even before the interview process, there should be goals set for the ministry to accomplish. Nurses are much more accustomed to working toward goals than most seminary-trained professionals. Those goals should be shared with the nurse during the interview process so that she will not be surprised the first day. Goals should be in writing so that there is a clear understanding of what is expected. Nurses have been taught to think, assess, plan, intervene, and evaluate. Having clear start-up goals will fit well into that type of thinking process.

The congregation needs to make space for the parish nurse, both physically and operationally. The parish nurse will need some physical space, such as an office that is close enough to the rest of the staff to allow collegial relationships with other staff, but private enough to allow confidential counseling with parishioners. Many parish nurses, however, have started out sharing a Sunday school room with the rest of the world. It is certainly not ideal, but parish nurses are generally resourceful and flexible people and this arrangement has worked.

The parish nurse also will need a desk, a locked file cabinet, a telephone, and a way to receive confidential messages. A computer with Internet access provides a definite advantage to his or her work, in that it allows for easy access to updated health information and efficient communication through e-mail. If possible, the office should be stocked with basic office supplies.

The health committee, in consultation with the pastor, must decide where the parish nurse will fit into the organizational chart of the congregation before the individual is offered the position. Who will be the immediate supervisor? Does the parish nurse report to a committee or board? Are written reports required on a regularly basis, and if so, how often—on a monthly or yearly basis? If these decisions can be made before the parish nurse begins it will help in getting the ministry started in the right direction.

The First Day

The member of the staff (usually the senior pastor) who will be the on-site supervisor should arrange some time the first day to meet with the parish nurse. This sets up the beginnings of a collegial relationship. If the parish nurse is not a member of the congregation, a tour of the facilities is a good way to spend some of that time. Be sure to arrange introductions to all other staff, including secretaries and custodians.

The pastor should explain some of the informal rules and rituals that every group has, such as what happens for lunch, how phone calls are handled, how and when others let the secretary know where they will be, and other little details that are important and trivial at the same time. The first day is a good time to arrange for regular meeting times. Nurses are accustomed to keeping their supervisors apprised of their progress. It will help the supervisor know if expected progress is being made toward goals and help keep little irritants from becoming huge problems.

It is also good for the pastor and parish nurse to set up an evaluation schedule. If working with a sponsoring institution, they will probably have an evaluation process. If not, does the congregation have a method of evaluating employees? If so, the parish nurse should be advised of the method and schedule. The pastor and parish nurse should also discuss any other policies, formal or informal, that may affect the work routine.

The parish nurse will then need some time to make the office comfortable. Time should be allocated for putting up pictures, rearranging the furniture, and learning the phone system.

The First Six Months

Clergy sometimes have a difficult time determining how to let the parish nurse perform a ministry that they have done in the past. One clergy person said, "I know just enough about medicine to be dangerous," but it is sometimes difficult to let that go. So it is important to psychologically make room for the parish nurse. During the first month, the pastor and parish nurse should arrange to make joint visits to the homebound and nursing home residents. They should work out a method of hospital visitation so that each does not show up at the same time.

The question should be addressed as to how the parish nurse will be notified of needs within the congregation/community. The parish nurse will also need to know how to make referrals to the clergy and how the clergy will refer parishioners or others to him or her. Getting all of these details worked out early will avoid confusion and hurt feelings later.

The pastor should discuss the procedure for scheduling educational programs, screenings, and support groups. For example, the parish nurse will need to know how rooms are reserved and whether or not programs need to be approved by the health cabinet, congregational governing body, or clergy. Getting these guidelines in place at the beginning will help the parish nurse determine how far in advance planning should begin. It will also help relationships with existing ministries.

The pastor will need to let the parish nurse know what support systems are in place to help the ministry. While we recommend that a parish nurse ministry not be started until a health cabinet is functioning, this does not always happen. In that case, the parish nurse should be assisted with assembling a health cabinet. Sometimes a health cabinet is already in place, but a health cabinet that convinced the congregation to initiate a health ministry does not necessarily have the right people to be a support system to a parish nurse. They may be visionaries, but what is needed next might be called "worker bees." A health cabinet full of visionaries may present the new parish nurse with too many good ideas or tasks but not want to help in the implementation. The congregation must be willing to accept the resignation of health cabinet members and assist in locating people who are willing to work with the parish nurse. There may be other groups that will also be supportive of the health ministry, such as parish visitors, education committees, outreach committees, and others. The parish nurse should meet with all boards and committees during the first six months but should start with those that are most related to a health ministry.

The parish nurse needs to be introduced to the congregation. There are a number of ways for this to happen, and it is best to use as many as possible. Parish nursing is often a quiet ministry and the congregation may wonder what is happening unless the ministry is made more visible.

If there is a bulletin board available, have the parish nurse post a picture and a short biographical sketch. Post the goals for the health ministry, as well as how to contact the parish nurse, and list the types of services the parish nurse will provide. In the newsletter, the parish nurse should write an introductory article with the same information that is posted on the bulletin board.

Business cards are essential for the parish nurse to give to parishioners and to leave when visiting in hospitals and nursing homes. Some churches have found brochures or flyers are helpful. The parish nurse can give them to people as she or he makes presentations to various committees and boards. A new logo for parish nursing is available through the International Parish Nurse Resource Center for use on business cards.

Recognition during worship is also important. Depending on the church's polity, there should be some type of service of installation (affirmation, dedication, commissioning), preferably during the first three months of the parish nurse's ministry there. If the church is in partnership with an institution, representatives from the institution should be included in the service. It may also be a good time to recognize the health cabinet and other health ministry volunteers. A sample service of installation is provided in appendix C.

If the person hired has not attended a parish nurse basic preparation course this should be accomplished within the first six months. This course provides essential information for establishing a parish nurse practice. It also offers an opportunity for the parish nurse to establish ties with other parish nurses. Nurses are accustomed to working with other nurses. Many find the parish a foreign culture, and having other nurses with whom to share joys and frustration is helpful. If there is a local or denominational network, encourage the parish nurse to be an active member.

Initial Programs

Usually one of the first programs a parish nurse establishes is blood pressure screening after worship. Screening gives the parish nurse an opportunity to meet a lot of parishioners. It also establishes the health ministry as a tool for health promotion and disease prevention. The congregation should supply the parish nurse with recently calibrated blood pressure equipment that includes three sizes of cuffs, a stethoscope, consent forms, and blood pressures cards to give to parishioners. Most parish nurses do this once a month and a regular group develops over a period of time. This can become a highly visible, easily recognizable service that can be used by many parishioners.

Other programs are more dependent on needs and goals of the program. If a health needs assessment was not done as part of the decision making process, it should be done now.[1] Needs assessment involves four steps. The first is to simply observe the environment both of the church and the community. This might involve a walking or driving tour of the neighborhood. The next step is to examine records. In the congregation this might involve annual reports, a pictorial directory, special services records, and so forth. In the community this would involve reports generated by the health department, community groups, or foundations. The third step is to interview key informants. Besides the clergy, the church secretary, chairpersons of all boards and committees, and informal church leaders should be interviewed. In the community, interviews should be sone with representatives of health care providers, emergency services providers, and social service agencies. The last step is to survey church members and/or communities and groups the ministry is to serve.

A survey can serve many different purposes. If one is undertaken in the first six months it should be seen as a way of introducing the parish nurse. Constructing a survey is not an easy task. If someone in the congregation has experience in constructing surveys, his or her help should be sought. Never put a service or topic on a survey that you are not prepared to attempt to address. How surveys are distributed depends on the size of the congregation. Having them completed during worship will yield the highest rate of return but will only reach regular worshippers. Mailing is expensive, and a 30 percent return rate would be considered excellent.

The positive thing about doing a survey early on is that many people in the congregation can have input in the direction of the health ministry. The most negative thing is setting unrealistic expectations by offering too many choices. The parish nurse program should be developed based on the needs identified in the health needs assessment. It is usually best to start with small programs such as a one-time education program and build on those successes. A sample health needs survey for a congregation can be found in appendix B.

The roles of referral agent and advocate should also be established in the first six months. The pastor can help by referring people who approach him or her with health concerns to the parish nurse. If the parish nurse can help members of the congregation, especially influential ones, to better utilize the health-care or social service system, it will generate great word of mouth publicity for the ministry.

Plans for the Future

Be aware that no ministry is built in a day. Even Jesus needed three years with the disciples to get the ministry going! A parish nurse should be given no less time. It takes time and perseverance to get a new ministry started. The pastor and congregation must assist in any way possible, including letting the parish nurse know that she or he is not alone. Be sure to include the parish nurse in all staff meetings and gatherings. This is especially important if the position is unpaid. Arrange at least one staff meeting a month that the parish nurse can attend.

In the middle of the third year, the congregation may wish to consider doing an effectiveness survey. One is available through the International Parish Nurse Resource Center.[2] This will help the congregation evaluate this new ministry. It also helps to obtain funding either from donors or outside sources.

Parish nursing is rapidly growing. It is an exciting new field of ministry. But like all things young it takes nurturing. The parish nurse will need direction, encouragement to continue growing, especially in developing spiritual care skills, and a chance to make mistakes. Not every program will be successful, but the learning from it will be invaluable.

Soon the parish nurse who did not know what to do on the first day will be asking, "How will I get it all done?" Health ministry is needed everywhere, within the congregation, in the community, and among the church staff. Parish nursing can play a vital role in addressing the wholistic health concerns of a community.

14

Parish Nurse Programming
An Abundance of Possibilities

I DEAS FOR PARISH NURSE PROGRAMMING are limited only by the imagination of the parish nurse and congregation working together on health ministry—in essence, the sky is the limit! Networking with other clergy and parish nurses will help the parish nurse discover more ideas. Looking at leading health indicators, such as those compiled by Healthy People 2010, might help identify some areas in which he or she may want to try to impact the health of the congregation and community. (Information about Healthy People 2010 is included in appendix G, "Parish Nurse Resources.")

Here are a few ideas for the parish nurse to consider as he or she begins to plan programming within the congregation and community.

Health Assessment

Parish nurses spend a great deal of their time assessing the health of the community, and they do this in a variety of ways, both on a micro and a macro level. The most common way of doing health assessment is through arranging for health screenings, which may be something as simple as regular blood pressure screenings after worship or as comprehensive as an annual health fair with a number of different screenings available. Some screenings arranged by parish nurses can be offered at no charge, others may necessitate a small fee. The parish nurse will want to arrange for the appropriate organization to do screenings. Clearly, a parish nurse is not qualified to administer a mammogram, nor would it fall within the scope and standards of his or her practice. Generally, though, these are the type of screenings that a parish nurse is easily able to provide or arrange through another organization:

1. blood pressure
2. blood sugar
3. cholesterol
4. mental health conditions, such as depression
5. bone density
6. vision and hearing
7. lung function
8. mammograms
9. lead poisoning
10. PSA testing (prostate cancer screening)

Parish nurses also may do a great deal of health assessment in their regular interactions with parishioners and members of the community, as they listen closely for clues about health concerns and issues. On a macro level, they may also arrange for data collection and analysis on health issues related to the entire congregation and/ or community in order to help design appropriate interventions, which may include parish nurse programming, or connection with other resources.

Health Education

Parish nurses provide health education through a variety of formats— through mission moments in church, newsletter articles, displays on bulletin boards, arranging for speakers and facilitators such as exercise class leaders, and meeting with individual parishioners to discuss specific health concerns.

Here are some ideas on health education topics to get a health cabinet started thinking about ways in which a parish nurse program might be helpful:

1. The parish nurse might teach a class on weight loss and nutrition. Sometimes a weight-loss program provided in an atmosphere where God's love and acceptance is shared is more successful than a simple "count your calories" program.

2. A qualified exercise instructor, who could teach an aerobics (or other form of exercise) class appropriate to the level of those wishing to participate, might be engaged by the parish nurse. There are exercise options appropriate to all ages, including the frail elderly who could benefit from armchair exercises.

3. The parish nurse might arrange for educational classes and support for new parents who might be isolated from extended family.

4. Parishioners who have specific health education questions, such as how to manage chronic diabetes or asthma, may meet with the parish nurse.

5. The parish nurse might arrange for other health professionals to speak with members of the congregation. For example, a cardiologist may talk about heart disease to a couple's group, or a dentist might address the important of dental hygiene to the children and their parents at Vacation Bible School.

6. CPR and first aid classes can be taught by a qualified instructor, which may be especially helpful for Sunday school teachers, daycare teachers, and nursery attendants.

7. Parenting classes may be developed, especially for parents of teenagers or other children presenting challenges.

8. The parish nurse may teach a class on women's health issues, such as breast cancer, osteoporosis, heart disease, and menopause.

9. Educational pieces for the newsletter about topics such as skin cancer, sexual abuse, domestic violence, mental health, meal planning for diabetics, fire safety, home safety, hospice, or other health-related issues may be written by the parish nurse.

10. The parish nurse may arrange for someone living with a specific health concern to make a presentation to a group within the congregation. Sometimes it is more helpful to hear from someone living with a disease, such as a survivor of breast cancer, than it is to hear from a health-care provider.

Health Advocacy

Health advocacy is a role that is often feared by parish nurses and congregations alike because it brings to mind an adversarial type of person. However, Jesus was an "advocate" for those he met, and he calls us to advocate for one another as well. Here are some ways in which a parish nurse can offer health advocacy:

1. The parish nurse may speak out for services that are needed in a community. For example, many of the parish nurses in St. Louis are advocating for better access to dental services, and some of the parish nurses have been arranging for dental equipment to be delivered to organizations that can expand their capacity with more dental equipment in place.

2. The parish nurse may speak out for a patient who is not receiving needed services and help that person wend his or her way through a disjointed medical system.

3. The parish nurse may accompany a parishioner on a visit to a medical professional and help that person understand options for treatment.

4. A congregation may be encouraged by a parish nurse to work toward providing the kind of healthy environment that is needed in a community, for example, helping an inner-city congregation develop a safe play area for children who have no other place to play.

5. The parish nurse may help identify people who are falling through the cracks in ways that are not readily apparent to the health-care system. For example, several of the parish nurses in St. Louis have been working together to advocate for an after-school meal program at an inner-city school near their churches for children who have been seen "dumpster diving" for food after class has been dismissed for the day. Other parish nurses have helped families get immunizations who have not been able to enroll their children in school because they had not yet obtained their immunizations. They arrange for the families to get to the immunization clinics and then for the families to get their children enrolled in school. Advocacy for kids to get to school is a health issue!

6. The parish nurse may take part in advocacy efforts such as campaigns to get funds allocated for smoking cessation programs and health education programs to prevent children from beginning to smoke.

7. Parish nurses may support the efforts of local lawmakers to enforce laws related to the environment, such as cleaning up the lead-based paint in rental housing.

8. The parish nurse may advocate for a more healthful environment within the congregation, such as healthier food served at church functions, or more vacation time for the clergy and other church staff.

9. A parish nurse may facilitate inclusion of the mentally ill and other disabled individuals within the worship life of the congregation. Most churches are easily able to accommodate some differences, but others take more assistance. Sometimes a parish nurse is able to locate the assistance that makes that inclusion possible, such as an interpreter for the deaf.

10. The parish nurse may advocate for the homebound and help them to become more active in the church, as she is able to connect them with other caregivers within the congregation, as well as others in need, such as those in need of prayer.

Development of Support Groups

Parish nurses work in tandem with others in the community to provide healing environments for people facing health challenges in their lives, which often have spiritual and social components. One of the best arenas for promoting wholeness is in a supportive environment with others who share similar concerns. A parish nurse is able to develop support groups, using the resources of other professionals, which can meet in a caring congregational setting. Some examples of support groups that parish nurses have developed include the following:

1. Support groups have been started by parish nurses to support single parents or others facing special challenges raising their children, using the skills of counselors or therapists. Some parish nurses have connected with

"Parents Anonymous," which helps parents who may be at risk for abusing their children to learn positive family-building skills. Mary Ann Brischetto has started a "Positive Family Program" with this concept at St. Paul United Church of Christ in St. Louis.

2. Alzheimer's support groups have been started by parish nurses to help assist caregivers in living with a loved one with this isolating and devastating disease. A parish nurse is uniquely positioned to understand the living situation of a caregiver. He or she also may have known both the people living with the disease and their families for many years, giving her an advantage over those in the health field who may have only just met the family and who may not understand the full complement of their strengths and concerns.

3. Support groups for divorced parishioners and community members, which are led by trained mental health professionals, are often very helpful. Those who are divorcing often lose their church community as they restructure their social support, and a support group can be way for them to stay connected with others and realize that they are not alone.

4. Parkinson's support groups provide education and mutual support to people who have this disease or who are living with someone affected by its progress. This is a disease where great strides are being made related to medications and medical interventions, and the education and support gained in such a group can be invaluable to a parishioner. It is also a place where one can be fully, unconditionally accepted, no matter how advanced the disease.

5. Groups such as Alcoholics Anonymous, Al-Anon, and other twelve-step programs are very helpful in supporting someone who has a chemical addiction or who is living with someone facing that challenge. While the parish nurse would not facilitate such a support group, the parish nurse certainly should be aware of where these support groups are located and could make appropriate referrals, or help develop one at the congregation if that particular need is unmet within the community. Of course, the parish nurse should also be aware of all treatment options for someone who is chemically dependent.

6. Families who have one or more members with mental illness often benefit from a support group where they can meet with others who share their concerns and where they can hear educational programs related to their particular interests. There are a number of organizations, such as the National Alliance for the Mentally Ill, who can provide resources to a parish nurse in helping to develop an appropriate support group.

7. Some congregations have started support groups specifically for families who are grieving the loss of a child, a profoundly tragic experience, and one that affects the other children, as well as the parents and extended family. It is often far easier for a family to travel to a church to attend a support group than it is for them to go back to the hospital where the child may have died.

8. As Americans live longer, those who are retired no longer fit into one group. There are the "young old" (sixty-five to seventy-five years old or so), the "old" (seventy-five to eighty-five years old or so), and the "old old" (around eighty-five years and older). Parish nurses often find that these different groups need to meet separately, as they have separate concerns and interests, being essentially from different generations. Some parish nurses have started support groups, such as the "Vintage Journey" at St. Trinity Lutheran Church in St. Louis, where parish nurse Jane Hahn has one group of elderly meet to discuss their lives and put together memory books to share with families.

9. One of the most effective parts of any weight-loss program is the support that one gets from others. Weight-loss support groups are very common in churches with parish nurses, and the pastor often is one of the people who can benefit most, given all the challenges of potlucks and parishioner hospitality! There are a variety of weight-loss programs that work well in a church setting, a number of which have spiritual themes.

10. Someone once said, "Whenever I get the urge to exercise, I simply lie down until that urge goes away." Health behaviors are so hard to change—especially the sedentary lifestyle. Parish nurses have started many support groups in congregations across the country to get people moving,

especially walking groups. One recent survey done by the Deaconess Parish Nurse Ministries showed that because of parish nurses, more than 1,200 people exercised (in twenty-nine churches) over a three-month period, most of whom would not have exercised otherwise. What a tremendous contribution to the health of a community, if not even one other thing happened through a parish nurse ministry! The ability to change health behaviors through the parish nurse ministry is remarkable. It is remarkable, but not surprising, because it is based on the power of relationships. Support groups play a large role in developing those strong relationships.

Coordination of Volunteers

A parish nurse is never going to be able to significantly impact the health of a congregation or community alone. Any parish nurse is going to need well-trained volunteers who are committed to the same cause of healing and wholeness for the congregation and the community. Health ministry often involves the concept of "each one teach one" and then some! Here are some ideas for parish nurse programming, using volunteers to help with the health ministry:

1. Volunteers are critical to the success of programs such as health fairs. It simply is not possible to put on a health fair without a number of volunteers who are willing to help with the arrangements and logistics.

2. Volunteers can help with the support of those who need extra help because of health-related concerns. For example, Joyce Lony, the parish nurse at Eden United Church of Christ in Edwardsville, Illinois, is also the coordinator of the Faith in Action program known as the Volunteer Interfaith Caregivers, which trains and arranges for volunteers to provide care to people with health issues who are still living in their homes but in need of assistance, such as meals, companionship, and light housekeeping.

3. Parish nurses often work in tandem with other volunteer outreach ministries, such as Stephen Ministries, to provide support for health-related concerns among those with whom the Stephen Ministers are working.

4. Parish nurses often know the needs and abilities of those whom they visit and can link volunteers together in ways that are meaningful to both. For example, Faith Roberts, parish nurse coordinator at Carle Foundation Hospital in Urbana, Illinois, shared the story of a homebound woman who was quite depressed and angry. Faith asked the woman to make a casserole for a single mother with a new baby who had no family nearby to help her with the demands and stresses of a newborn. The homebound woman was able to provide meals, as well as moral support, to the younger woman, who ended up becoming friends with this formerly lonely parishioner and who brought her baby to visit often.

5. Volunteers can provide support to various parish nurse programs, such as refreshments or child care for a support group. Having the congregation provide a meal and child care for a parenting support class gives parents who are already feeling overwhelmed a small break to look forward to as part of this outreach ministry.

6. Volunteers can get the word out about parish nurse ministry and help with financial support. The more that parishioners feel tied into and included in a ministry, the more likely they are to want to be involved in supporting the program financially.

7. Volunteers can help recruit other volunteers for health-related programs. For example, a volunteer who is a platelet donor is much more likely to be able to recruit others to consider this important and life-saving form of volunteering than the parish nurse is able to do alone.

8. Volunteers can help to staff programs such as telephone trees that check in on the homebound on a regular basis. You do not need to be able to drive to make a phone call— this is a volunteer service that homebound people can do for others.

9. Volunteers can help get people out for screenings, such as mammograms, by talking frankly with their friends, who might be more willing to listen to them about personal health-related issues than they would a pastor, or even a parish nurse they don't know well.

10. Volunteers can help with sports programs for children and youth, many of whom are at risk for obesity. Clare Duffy, parish nurse at Ebenezer Lutheran Church (LCMS) in St. Louis, runs a day camp for inner-city children in her congregation's neighborhood. A large portion of the program is focused on sports and other physical activities, which promote the health of the youngsters involved.

It must be noted that all parish nurse programming must be infused with the integration of faith and health. Further, the health ministry of a congregation should not be seen as a "piece" of its work, but rather as an integral ingredient of the whole. Food at church gatherings should be healthy, the environment should be nurturing, and programming should always be designed with health in mind. To use a cooking analogy, parish nursing is not like a slice of cheese in a ham and cheese sandwich, but more like eggs in a quiche. It takes a while to cook up a delicious recipe for healthful congregational living, but it is worth the work and wait!

15

Making Health Ministry Accessible and Visible

The Health Fair

One of the first events that clergy and health cabinets with a new parish nurse want to see take place is a health fair. It is a great way to provide visibility for the parish nurse program and promote wellness and prevention within the congregation. However, a health fair must be carefully planned and executed. This chapter was written by Elizabeth Durban, R.N., who is the Deaconess parish nurse at St. Gabriel's Catholic Church in St. Louis. Beth has a strong track record of outstanding health fairs and shares some of her wisdom here.

HEALTH FAIRS ARE EXCELLENT projects to promote health awareness and they provide a wonderful opportunity for the parish nurse to reach out to the whole community. Health fairs, however, take considerable preparation, time, and knowledge of the resources available. It definitely is not something a new parish nurse should undertake the first year. Many parish nurses have found themselves hosting a health fair with more providers than visitors. A health fair takes far too much effort to end up with the parish nurse feeling like a failure, and it would be unfair to ask a parish nurse to initiate one too soon. Once he or she is established in the parish and aware of the health needs of the community and how best to minister to them, then it is time to begin planning a health fair.

Planning

The planning phase is a critical part of a successful health fair. Without a good plan, each step becomes more difficult and fragmented. Although a good plan does not ensure success, it may help avert disaster. The parish nurse and health cabinet should decide what they would like to accomplish through a health fair and then establish written goals and objectives. Starting the process about six to nine months in advance of the fair is wise.

Sample goals for your health fair might be to:

- increase health awareness
- provide a variety of health screenings, educational materials, and referrals to community resources
- motivate parishioners toward making positive health behavior changes

Sample objectives for a health fair might be to:

- provide a targeted number (perhaps ten) of booths on different health awareness topics
- have three components within each booth at the fair—education, experience, and excitement
- identify parishioners with a specific health challenge (for example, hypertension) and follow up on the findings

The goals and objectives selected will be used to evaluate the overall success of the health fair. A time line should be developed, so that each step can be taken at a slow pace, rather than a "panic run" at the last moment. In addition, it is better to start small with the first fair and expand the next time.

Content

The type and number of booths at the health fair is only limited by space, time, and imagination. The best health fairs have interactive, experiential, hands-on booths that give the participants the opportunity to get immediate feedback on health issues. These fairs have a variety of topics, samples, giveaways, and exciting, motivated health professionals delivering their messages. In general, the content of a health fair can be divided into three categories: awareness, screenings, and demonstrations/activities.

Awareness. Awareness and information booths should be interactive rather than a stack of brochures on a table. Some topics for awareness booths include: cancer, women's health, nutrition, bicycle safety, dental health, elder care resources, and stress management.

Screenings. At health fairs screenings are conducted to increase awareness of health risks. Participants enjoy the variety of screening tests, especially if they are designed to give immediate feedback. For example, participants are more likely to have their cholesterol levels checked at a health fair if they get the results in three minutes and have the opportunity to discuss the results with a health professional immediately. Most screenings take several minutes per person, so enough screeners should be scheduled to accommodate the expected participation without creating long waiting lines. The screening booths should also be located in such a way so that long lines do not interfere with other booths. Possible health fair screenings might include blood pressure, total cholesterol, vision testing, hearing tests, spinal screening, body fat measurement, or oral cancer screening.

Demonstrations. Demonstrations and health awareness activities can add life and variety to the health fair. The adult learning theory reminds us that a hands-on opportunity enhances awareness, so participation in a demonstration or activity can help promote positive health behavior changes. Possible demonstrations and activities might include topics such as upper body massage, proper lifting, yoga, healthy cooking demonstrations, an "Ask the Doctor" booth, or reflexology.

When and Where

Once the content of the health fair is decided, the date, time, and location are the next biggest decisions. Consider the time of year, the people that will be attending (congregation, community, children, adults), and the space available at the parish. As far as length of time for the fair, four hours is workable and adequate.

In general, it is probably best to schedule the health fair in the spring or fall months—avoid summer and holiday seasons when people are likely to be on vacation. For a community health fair, weekends seem to work better. Another consideration is whether other health-related events going on in the community might conflict. It never hurts to have the health fair coincide with another event at church, however, where people will already be around.

Walk through all possible locations for the health fair (buildings, cafeterias, parking lot, gym) to discover the best venue. A space large enough to safely accommodate the planned number of booths and to allow enough room for those attending to circulate will be needed. Ideally, the site will be in a central location and easily accessible. The area should be checked carefully to ensure that there are enough electrical outlets. If all the attendees are to register for the health fair, designate one main entrance where participants can be greeted as they enter. If the health fair is to be held outside, be sure to have a contingency plan for rain, wind, or extreme heat. Don't forget about electrical needs. If long extension cords must be used, be sure to tape them down.

The parish nurse should not do everything alone—that is what health cabinets and other volunteers are for. He or she should delegate! Delegate! Delegate! Each task should be clearly defined, with a time frame for expected completion. Many hands make light work and less frazzled parish nurses.

Get Started

Once the planning is complete, the implementation begins with contacting potential providers by phone. Six to nine months ahead may seem too early, but often providers book up months in advance. Calling the providers initially is much better than writing. They will need to know the basics—the date, time, location, anticipated number of participants, and what is expected of them. The advantage of contacting providers first by telephone is that the parish nurse is able to field concerns and questions immediately and ascertain whether the provider will or will not participate. If one sounds doubtful about participating, the next choice of provider for a similar service should be contacted. If a provider sounds interested in helping, a verbal commitment should be obtained, followed up with a confirmation letter from the parish nurse. The letter should include a form, which requests any needed information by a specific date. Incidentally, other parish nurses are excellent resources for names of providers that they have found useful. They can share what has worked or not worked for them.

Almost every community has voluntary agencies that could participate in a health fair. If the voluntary agency is not able to send an excellent, experienced volunteer with some type of interactive display to the fair, they should be thanked but not invited to attend. More is not necessarily better. A few staffed booths will provide a much better health fair than thirty booths stacked high with pamphlets and no one sitting behind the table. There is nothing exciting about walking around a room just picking up brochures, and a boring event will make the parishioners think twice before returning for another fair. Make the fair enjoyable and a learning experience at the same time.

Providers can educate participants about their particular areas. They can also be invaluable sources of free information, screenings, and giveaways. Providers should be asked if they could supply an attendance prize.

A good, consistent theme throughout the health fair can tie the event together and make the event more fun and memorable. Having a theme affords continuity for decorations, learning opportunities, and the overall success of the health fair. Your theme may be based on other events, including seasonal holidays or national health observances. For example, if your health fair is in February, you might consider a Valentine's heart theme, especially because it is also National Heart Month. Other themes based on the time of year might be "Healthy Wintertime Fun," "Spring into Health," or "Fall into Fitness." A theme for a family-oriented health fair might be, "A Family Af-Fair."

One savvy parish nurse with a great deal of familiarity with the community in which she served knew that there were a large number of children from economically challenged families living nearby. As part of the health fair for her congregation, she arranged for book bags and school supplies to be distributed, as well as for a barber and beautician to be on hand. She attracted the kids, got them ready for school, and did health assessments on the side. That congregation's health fair was a huge success, because she did her homework to discern what that neighborhood really needed.

Freebies

One way to get people to attend a health fair is to offer "freebies." These freebies include items such as food samples, mugs, pens, toothbrushes, sunscreen samples, writing pads—the possibilities are limitless. Many organizations are happy to provide free products or samples to give out at the health fair. This provides some publicity for them and doesn't break the health fair budget.

If there are drug representatives in the congregation, they may be able to supply some giveaways. The number of items that they can provide free for such a purpose is surprising. The key is *free*. Requests for donations should be typed on church stationery and can be sent by health cabinet members. Grocery stores may donate fruit to use as refreshments for the fair. Great health fairs can be planned using a shoestring budget. Just get out there, make contacts, and don't be afraid to ask.

Promotion

The best way to ensure good attendance at a health fair is to promote, promote, promote! The health fair theme should be used to maintain consistency on all promotional material. Visibility is vital. If someone in the parish is experienced in public relations, by all means solicit his or her help. Getting articles in newspapers, announcements on the radio, flyers posted, and any other forms of publicity are all great for promoting the fair. A few months in advance, a message should be placed in the church bulletin or newsletter, letting everyone know that a special event is coming and asking them to save the date. As the date gets closer—about a month before—put more information in the bulletin elevating awareness of all that will happen that day. If there is a school with the church, send flyers home with the children. Word of mouth is a very effective method of promotion as well. Encourage the health cabinet, friends, and anyone else to "talk up" the health fair to the community.

The week before the fair a *very important* thing to do is for the parish nurse to call all the providers that will be at the fair. It reminds them and they can inform the congregation if they have changed their plans about attending. This reduces the chances of getting to the day and seeing empty tables because providers did not show up.

Floor Plan

It is best to design a floor plan or layout depicting the booth and provider set-up. When designing the layout, keep the following in mind:

Space. Some providers will need a small space and some might have an elaborate set-up. Let providers know how much space they can have, and make sure they inform the planners in advance of their requirements.

Electricity. If a provider needs electricity, place that booth as close as possible to an outlet to minimize safety hazards.

Traffic flow. Some booths may be very popular (screening tests) and cause lines to form. These booths may need more space or placement next to less popular booths. People then might look closely at the less popular booth while waiting in line.

Registration. Having the participants register for the health fair serves two purposes: it provides an accurate count of attendees, and it provides names from which to draw for the attendance prizes.

Last Minute "To Do" List

The parish nurse should make a checklist of all the supplies, materials, literature, and goodies gathered over the last few months. Everything should be assembled in one place to prevent anything from being forgotten. It is wise to make up an emergency kit with all kinds of general supplies. A provider may forget something, and the parish nurse will be the hero when he or she reaches into a box and comes up with the item to solve the problem. It also saves running around at the last minute trying to help providers.

Almost There

If at all possible, the health fair should be set up the night before. Hint: If helium balloons are used, wait to blow them up—they may be floating on the floor in the morning! If it is not possible to set up the night before, the parish nurse and some of the volunteers should get there *early*—at least two hours before the event.

Make sure providers arrive at least thirty minutes in advance so they can set up before the fair begins without a last-minute panic. Providers should be greeted as they arrive and thanked for their participation. They should then be directed to their respective tables, each of which has a card on it with the organization's or provider's name.

At the appointed hour, the parish nurse and health cabinet should take a deep breath, open the doors, and enjoy. This is their opportunity to meet people in the community and to promote parish nursing.

Wrap It Up

The health cabinet and all the volunteers need to be thanked for their hard work in making the health fair a success. Within a week or so after the fair, the parish nurse should also send a thank-you note to each of the providers, in which some of the results of the health fair can be shared. They gave the congregation a valuable service and deserve some recognition.

Last but not least, the parish nurse should compile all the health fair information into one folder. It will be a great resource for the next health fair. All correspondence, forms, sales receipts, notes, public relations information, provider names and addresses, and anything else that will be beneficial for the next fair should be included.

With proper planning, content, scheduling, and implementation, a health fair can be hosted successfully. It is hard work but a very rewarding experience!

Final Word

PARISH NURSING IS AN AMAZING ministry and practice, which is growing and evolving rapidly. It is currently ahead of the curve in ecumenical relationships and opening doors in interfaith partnerships as well. It is also ahead of the curve in forging relationships between nurses in nations around the world.

Through relationships, parish nurses, more than most other health-care providers, have the opportunity to change health behaviors at rates far higher than is possible in other settings. The church, with no fees or premiums charged for parish nurse services, is uniquely positioned to open doors for people who have been shut out from care for too long—people who are distrustful of the health-care system, people who are too poor to be of interest to the revenue-seeking providers, and people who are not on anyone's radar screen because they are not necessarily perceived to be at risk.

Parish nursing is about health for the whole body of Christ, for the whole community, indeed, for the world. It is a ministry that is essential today, for parishioners, for congregations, and for communities. It is my hope and prayer that you will carefully consider parish nursing as a ministry in your congregation.

Appendix A
Sample Parish Nurse Job Description

Job title: parish nurse

Supervised by: (title of parish nurse program coordinator/manager/director or pastor)

Job classification: exempt

All duties and standards of this position will be performed according to established policies, procedures, and guidelines for (name of sponsoring organization). These examples of work are not all-encompassing or restrictive and are expected to vary with changing needs and priorities. The duties for a specific position with this title will be defined and assigned by the site supervisor.

Statement of Purpose

The parish nurse is responsible for working in consultation with the (title of parish nurse program coordinator/manager/director), in accordance with a covenantal agreement between (sponsoring organization) and the church/agency. The parish nurse plays a highly visible role in the life and activities of the congregation/community to which assigned, while actively participating in the mission interpretation and promotion of the parish nursing ministry.

Job Duties and Responsibilities

I. Integrator of Faith and Health
Seeks to promote an understanding of the relationship between faith and health by:

    A. lifting up lifestyle practices as a matter of stewardship and faith

B. participating in the worship life of the faith community

C. providing spiritual care and guidance surrounding health issues

II. Health Educator

Provides health education in the congregation and community by:

A. coordinating and/or presenting health related classes or courses

B. securing guest presenters for special courses

C. providing articles for the church bulletin, newsletter, or other publication as requested

D. maintaining a health ministry bulletin board and/or literature rack at the church

E. arranging for use of church facilities as appropriate for health education activities

III. Health Counselor

Acts as a health consultant by:

A. wholistically assessing individuals in their homes and within the congregational setting

B. assessing the health of the congregation and wider community and developing appropriate programming to address health-related needs

C. accepting appropriate referrals

D. providing health screenings

E. assisting with visitation and follow up in homes, hospitals and long-term care facilities

IV. Referral Advisor

Acts as a referral source for members of the congregation and/or community served by:

A. referring individuals to pastor, physician, or community support services as needed

B. acting as a liaison between congregation and community resources

C. maintaining an awareness of the resources within the community

V. Health Advocate

Acts as a health advocate by:

A. assisting people to understand and effectively use health care and social service systems

B. serving as a resource person to other church committees and community organizations on health issues as requested

C. making the church staff and congregation aware of social and/or legislative issues that affect health care

VI. Developer of Support Groups

Acts as a developer of support groups by:

A. assessing the need for support groups in various health-related areas

B. facilitating the development of support groups for the faith community and others served, as needed

C. arranging for appropriate professional leadership for support groups as required

D. evaluating effectiveness of support groups in meeting health-related needs of participants

VII. Health Ministry Volunteer Coordinator

Coordinates health ministry volunteer activity (may include student nurses or paid staff) by:

A. recruiting volunteers for various health ministry activities

B. providing orientation and continuing education for volunteers

C. directing volunteer activities

D. evaluating volunteer performance and providing appropriate feedback and recognition

VIII. Collegiality

Maintains a positive working relationship with others by:

A. participating in regular meetings with the parish pastor and staff

B. meeting with and providing staff support for the health cabinet or advisory board

C. actively participating in the meetings called by the (sponsoring organization)

D. participating in the local parish nurse network or other professional organization

IX. Education

Acquires and maintains current knowledge in nursing practice, health promotion, and spiritual care by:

A. participating in continuing education in-service programs and other educational activities authorized by the congregation and (sponsoring organization)

B. attending any program deemed mandatory by the (sponsoring organization)

X. Quality Assurance

Systematically participates in evaluation of quality and effectiveness of practice by:

A. evaluating the program on a continuing basis with appropriate parties

B. providing the congregation and (sponsoring organization) with appropriate statistical data in a timely fashion

C. documenting services provided according to congregation and/or (sponsoring organization) requirements

D. participating in quality assurance activities initiated by the congregation or (sponsoring organization)

Job Requisites

A. Education and Training

1. graduate from an accredited School of Nursing

2. B.S.N. preferred

3. C.P.E. or theological education helpful

B. Licensing/Registration/Certification

    1. currently licensed as a registered nurse in the state of (name of state in which congregation is located)

    2. minimum of three years of experience, preferably in one or more of the following areas: public health, health education, public school nursing, medical/surgical and/or emergency room outpatient nursing

C. Skills and Abilities

    1. Excellent communication skills and teaching techniques

    2. Knowledge of current nursing and health-care issues in health promotion as related to lifestyle

    3. Knowledge of health services and resources in community

    4. Demonstrated knowledge of organizational dynamics of the denomination to be served

    5. Excellent organizational skills

    6. Participation in church and community activities that contribute to professional growth and to promotion of wholistic health philosophy

An individual without the requisites stated above may present a written justification explaining the relevance of his or her background for this position. Depending on organizational needs and availability of more qualified applicants, an applicant may have some or all requisites revised or waived.

Physical Requirements/Working Conditions

    1. manual dexterity, coordination, and skillful use of hands for working with required equipment

    2. ability to receive and express detailed information through oral communication, visual acuity, and the ability to read and understand written direction

    3. ability to physically perform necessary documentation in writing or through use of tape recorder

4. ability to occasionally lift and transport items weighing up to 10 pounds

Machines/Equipment/Tools

1. primary: telephone, information system with the parish
2. motor vehicle for travel within the community
3. secondary: fax, copy machine

Employee Acknowledgement

I have reviewed and I understand the job duties and expectations outlined in this job description.

I agree to perform the work in a manner acceptable to my immediate supervisor and within guidelines defined by the (sponsoring organization).

I also understand that continued employment will depend on my demonstrated ability to perform the work as expected.

Employee_____ Date_____

Appendix B

Sample Congregational Health Needs Survey

THE HEALTH CABINET OF (name of congregation) is seeking your opinions on the health needs of our congregation and community. We are collecting this information in order to help plan the programs and priorities for our new parish nurse ministry.

As you know, the roles of a parish nurse are to function in the following capacities: integrator of faith and health, health educator, health counselor, referral advisor, health advocate, developer of support groups, and volunteer coordinator. Please answer the questions below and check all items that apply.

Thank you!

Check the topics you would like to see as part of the parish nurse ministry programming.

1. ❑ nutrition

2. ❑ exercise

3. ❑ smoking, alcohol, drugs

4. ❑ stress management

5. ❑ disease management:

    a. ❑ AIDS

    b. ❑ diabetes

    c. ❑ heart disease

    d. ❑ stroke recovery

    e. ❑ other (please specify):_____

6. ❑ relationships

7. ❑ parenting

8. ❑ infant care

9. ❑ CPR/first aid

10. ❑ sexuality

11. ❑ men's health issues

12. ❑ women's health issues

13. ❑ mental health issues

14. ❑ domestic violence

15. ❑ dental health

16. ❑ safety

17. ❑ spiritual topics

18. ❑ hospice, end-of-life issues

19. ❑ insurance/Medicare/Medicaid

20. ❑ other (please specify):_____

Do you see a need for health events in the congregation? If so, which should be started (or continued)?

1. ❑ blood drives

2. ❑ health screenings:

    a. ❑ blood pressure

    b. ❑ cholesterol

    c. ❑ diabetes

    d. ❑ mental health screenings

    e. ❑ bone density

    f. ❑ vision

    g. ❑ hearing

    h. ❑ lung function

     i. ❑ mammograms

     j. ❑ PSA testing (prostate cancer screening)

     k. ❑ dental screening

     l. ❑ lead poisoning

3. ❑ healing service

4. ❑ flu shots

5. ❑ other (please specify):_____

Do you see a need for support groups in the congregation? If so, which should be started (or continued)?

1. ❑ twelve-step groups, such as Alcoholics Anonymous, Alanon, Alateen, Narcotics Anonymous, and Overeaters Anonymous
Please specify: _____

2. ❑ caregivers support

3. ❑ divorce support

4. ❑ grief support

5. ❑ parenting support

6. ❑ exercise club

7. ❑ weight management

8. ❑ pain management support
(arthritis, osteoporosis, back pain, etc.)

9. ❑ adoption support group

10. ❑ asthma support group

11. ❑ other (please specify):_____

In your opinion, the parish nurse should:

1. ❑ serve the congregation only.

2. ❑ serve the surrounding community only.

3. ❑ serve both the congregation and the community.

4. ❑ provide educational health moments in the worship service.

5. ❑ provide educational health materials in the bulletin.

6. ❑ provide educational health materials in the newsletter.

7. ❑ provide educational health materials on a bulletin board.

8. ❑ provide health counseling to individuals.

9. ❑ arrange for health screenings at the church.

10. ❑ arrange for dental screenings at the church.

11. ❑ visit the hospitalized.

12. ❑ visit the homebound.

13. ❑ visit new mothers.

14. ❑ provide spiritual support.

15. ❑ make the congregation aware of social and/or legislative health-care issues.

16. ❑ refer to appropriate community and/or medical services as needed.

Please answer these questions about yourself in relation to the parish nurse ministry. "I would like . . ."

1. ❑ to talk to the parish nurse about health concerns.

2. ❑ to talk to the parish nurse about my diet.

3. ❑ to talk to the parish nurse about health concerns of family members.

4. ❑ the parish nurse to be able to assist me in crisis situations.

5. ❑ the parish nurse to be able to advocate for me in the health care system.

6. ❑ the parish nurse to go with me to the doctor.

7. ❑ the parish nurse to go with me if I need surgery.

8. ❑ the parish nurse to visit me if I were hospitalized.

9. ❑ to participate in an parish nurse-sponsored exercise program.

10. ❑ to attend health-related parish nurse educational programs.

11. ❑ to participate in health screenings at our church.

12. ❑ to volunteer to help with the parish nurse program.

Comments:

Thank you for your time and suggestions!

The Health Cabinet, (name of congregation).

Please note:
These questions may also be used as a telephone survey for the homebound.

Appendix C
Sample Service of Installation for a Parish Nurse

Order of Worship

Prelude

Welcome and Greetings

Call to Worship

Leader: God calls forth life from the waters of the earth, and healing from springs of eternal love.

People: We worship the God who has made us whole— body, mind and spirit—and placed us as stewards of all the earth.

Leader: We sing praise to God because we are grateful for God's faithfulness in trial and rejoicing.

People: There is nowhere we can go from God's presence. God comes to us with compassionate, strengthening love.

Leader: God calls us to respond with courage and steadfastness, as partners in bringing hope and peace to the world.

People: Let us wosrship together the God who has made us whole, forgiven our sins, and graced us with talents and challenges.

Opening Hymn—Suggested Hymns:

"Joyful, Joyful, We Adore You"
Tune: Hymn to Joy, Beethoven, 1824
Text: Henry van Dyke, 1907

"Sing Praise to God, Our Highest Good"
Tune: Mit Freuden Zart,
Bohemian Brethren's Kirchengesang, 1566
Text: Johann J. Schutz, 1675

"Bring Many Names"
Tune: Westchase, Carlton Young, 1989
Text: Brian Wren, 1989

Greetings and Congratulations

(Greetings may come from the organization sponsoring the parish nurse program, from a denominational representative, or from a parish nurse in a neighboring congregation or community.)

Pastor: Today, we celebrate and proclaim the covenant of ministry between our parish nurse (name), (name of congregation), and (name of organization sponsoring parish nurse program). (Name of individual) will represent (sponsoring organization) in the proclamation of this covenant.

A Covenant and Affirmation of Ministry

A Time of Covenant Making

Church Representative: Life takes on richer meaning, greater depth, and faithful direction when covenants are boldly proclaimed and affirmed in God's presence.

People: **We stand before God, as people with whom God has made covenants. We covenant this day with (name of parish nurse), and with the staff of (name of sponsoring organization) to support, expand, and convey our commitment to God's healing and eternal love.**

We commit ourselves to better understand, reflect, and convey God's will for all of God's children to live abundantly through God's amazing grace. May we live boldly in the presence of God!

Church Representative: (Name of parish nurse), as a parish nurse at (name of congregation), what are you prepared to contribute, share, and commit to within this new health ministry?

Parish Nurse: I will attempt to follow God's will and to work with the pastor(s) and congregation in my parish nursing efforts. In times of both trauma and joy, I will persistently try to proclaim and trust the healing power of God's love for the members of this congregation and for the people of this community.

Church Representative: (Name of organizational representative), as a representative of (sponsoring organization), what are you prepared to contribute, share, and commit in this new health ministry?

Representative from Sponsoring Organization: We will help generate financial support for this parish nurse program, and we will provide ongoing guidance, education, and support in order to enrich and expand the already existing talents and education of (name of parish nurse). We will work with the leaders and members of (name of church) to help ensure that this ministry will reach beyond the local church membership and impact the health and wholeness of its neighbors.

All: **Bless this covenant, O God, and walk with us as we strive to be faithful sojourners in your way. As we travel, help us to grow in stamina, wisdom, love, and faith. Amen.**

Scripture Lesson

Hymn or Anthem[1]

Sermon

Pastoral Prayer and Lord's Prayer

Offertory

*Presentation of Offerings

Doxology: **Praise God from whom all blessing flow;**
Praise Christ the Word in flesh born low;
Praise Holy Spirit evermore;
One God, Triune, whom we adore.[2]

*Prayer of Thanksgiving

All: **O God of peace and God of wisdom, we rejoice and**
give thanks for the ministry of (name of parish
nurse) among us and with us. We pray that you
will use each of us to bring healing and wholeness
to the world. For the ways you lead us and bless us
as we seek to bring your love to all people, we say,
Amen.

*Closing Hymn

"In Our Hearts and Neighborhoods"[3]
Suggested tune: Royal Oak ("All Things Bright and Beautiful")
7.6.7.6 with refrain
Text: Deborah Patterson, c. 1996

Refrain: **In our hearts and neighborhoods**
we sow the seeds of peace.
We would plant community,
love's harvest to increase.

We work for hope and healing.
We seek the lonely soul.
We stretch out hands in friendship,
that God might make us whole. (*Refrain*)

We pray for all the children,
for youth who need our care,
for lonely homebound elders
with gifts they long to share. (*Refrain*)

Oh, send us forth in courage,
equipped with grace to know
diversity's rich garden,
God's love and care to grow. *(Refrain)*

Benediction

Postlude

indicates that the congregation should stand

Appendix D
Sample Parish Nurse Survey for the Congregation

W E WOULD LIKE YOUR INPUT about the parish nurse health ministry of our congregation. *Please circle the response* that best describes your feelings about the following statements:

1. Our congregation is becoming comfortable with the idea that a person's health results from the interaction between behaviors, attitudes, faith, and beliefs.

    Yes   No

2. Health and healing are becoming more important parts of our church's mission and everyday activities.

    Yes   No

3. I have read bulletins and newsletter articles on health topics provided by the parish nurse.

    Yes   No

4. I have participated in health screenings, health fairs, educational programs, or support groups offered by the parish nurse program.

    Yes   No

5. I have talked with the parish nurse about a health matter such as medication, a diagnosis or health condition, a relationship, or my overall health and well-being.

    Yes   No

6. I know someone who has talked with the parish nurse about a health matter.

    Yes   No

7. The parish nurse has referred me to a physician, a group, or an organization in the congregation or community where I could go for further assistance.

   Yes   No

8. I have changed my lifestyle as a result of the parish nurse program.

   Yes   No

9. I have participated in a ministry from this congregation that provides services to the poor, homeless, homebound, or bereaved in cooperation with the parish nurse program.

   Yes   No

10. A church volunteer has provided support to me during a time of personal need.

    Yes   No

11. The parish nurse has provided support to me or my family that helped me/us draw upon my/our spiritual strength in dealing with health issues.

    Yes   No

12. The parish nurse program offers a variety of support services and activities to our congregation. How familiar are you with the parish nurse program here?

    Very familiar

    Somewhat familiar

    Not at all familiar

13. When you have a health question or crisis where do you get support or information?

14. Circle the letter in front of each activity you would like the parish nurse program to continue or begin:

    a. articles on health topics in bulletins and newsletters

    b. health screening activities

c. health education programs or support groups

d. information on other community groups, organizations, and services

e. opportunities to participate as a part of the health ministry

f. opportunities to discuss the relationship between my faith and health

g. visiting members who are homebound, hospitalized, or in long-term care facilities

h. other (please specify):

15. Circle all appropriate responses:

My age group:

13–17	18–30	31–50
51–65	66–80	80+

I am: female   male

I am: single   married   separated

divorced   widowed

I am a member of this church:

Yes   No

16. I am willing to support the parish nurse program through (circle the letter before each item that applies):

a. volunteering my time and talents

b. sharing my financial support

c. lifting up the ministry in prayer

17. I believe the program should continue.

Yes   No

Need more information to decide

Please use this space to provide comments on parish nurse program:

If you were the parish nurse, what would you do differently?

Appendix E

Sample Parish Nurse Performance Evaluation Tool

Employee name_____

Employee social security number_____

Scheduled review date_____

❑ Six-month review ❑ Annual review (*Check one*)

Overall rating_____
(See performance rating levels below—exceeds, meets, does not meet standards)

Purpose

The purpose of the performance review is for the pastor/supervisor, director/manager, and parish nurse to thoroughly review the parish nurse's past performance and develop goals and objectives for the coming year.

Performance Rating Levels

The following performance levels should be used to rate the parish nurse's level of performance with regard to each duty:

Frequently exceeds standard. The standard is frequently (more often than not) exceeded. The level of performance is clearly and substantially above what is required. The parish nurse shows a clear understanding of all functions of the particular duty. The results achieved are better than expected as standard.

Meets standard. The standard is met. The level of performance meets the standard requirement of the position. Assignments are performed in an acceptable manner.

Does not meet standard. The standard is not always met. The level of performance is generally below what is expected, showing need for improvement. The pastor/supervisor, director/manager, and parish nurse must agree on a plan of action for improvement, set goals, and establish a date by which progress is to be achieved.

Procedures

One month before the performance review is due, the director/manager of the parish nurse program will give the parish nurse two evaluation forms. One is to be completed by the pastor/supervisor and the other is to be used as a self-evaluation. Each subcategory is rated and from this an overall rating for each category is determined.

An evaluation session is then scheduled with the director/manager of parish nursing. During this session the final ratings and comments are determined.

The form is then signed by the pastor/supervisor, director/manager, and parish nurse. Copies will be made and distributed to all parties. The original is kept on file in the office of the director of parish nursing.

The amount of salary increase will be based on the evaluation and budgetary constraints at both the church and parish nurse program.

Performance Level Scoring

INTEGRATOR OF FAITH AND HEALTH

	Exceeds	Meets	Does not meet
E			
P/S			
F			

(*E=employee, P/S=pastor/supervisor, F=final scoring)

Seeks to promote an understanding of the relationship between faith and health by:

    a. lifting up lifestyle practices as a matter of stewardship and faith

    b. participating in the worship life of the faith community

    c. providing spiritual care and guidance surrounding health issues

Comments:

HEALTH EDUCATOR

	Exceeds	Meets	Does not meet
E			
P/S			
F			

(*E=employee, P/S=pastor/supervisor, F=final scoring)

Provides health education in the congregation and community by:

    a. coordinating and/or presenting health related classes or courses

    b. securing guest presenters for special courses

    c. providing articles for the church bulletin, newsletter or other publications as requested

    d. maintaining a health ministry bulletin board and/or literature rack at the church

    e. arranging for use of church facilities as appropriate for health education activities

Comments:

HEALTH COUNSELOR

	Exceeds	Meets	Does not meet
E			
P/S			
F			

(*E=employee, P/S=pastor/supervisor, F=final scoring)

Acts as a health consultant by:

    a. wholistically assessing individuals in their homes and within the congregational setting

    b. assessing the health of the congregation and wider community and developing appropriate programming to address health-related needs

    c. accepting appropriate referrals

    d. providing health screenings

    e. assisting with visitation and follow-up in homes, hospitals, and long-term care facilities

Comments:

REFERRAL ADVISOR

	Exceeds	Meets	Does not meet
E			
P/S			
F			

(*E=employee, P/S=pastor/supervisor, F=final scoring)

Acts as a referral source for members of the congregation and/or community served by:

a. referring individuals to pastor, physician, or community support services as needed

b. acting as a liaison between congregation and community resources

c. maintaining an awareness of the resources within the community

Comments:

HEALTH ADVOCATE

	Exceeds	Meets	Does not meet
E			
P/S			
F			

(*E=employee, P/S=pastor/supervisor, F=final scoring)

Acts as a health advocate by:

a. assisting people to understand and effectively use health care and social service systems

b. serving as a resource person to other church committees and to community organizations on health issues as requested

c. making the church staff and congregation aware of social and/or legislative issues that affect health care

Comments:

DEVELOPER OF SUPPORT GROUPS

	Exceeds	Meets	Does not meet
E			
P/S			
F			

(*E=employee, P/S=pastor/supervisor, F=final scoring)

Acts as a developer of support groups by:

   a. assessing the need for support groups in various health-related areas

   b. facilitating the development of support groups for the faith community and others served, as needed

   c. arranging for appropriate professional leadership for support groups as required

   d. evaluating effectiveness of support groups in meeting health-related needs of participants

Comments:

HEALTH MINISTRY VOLUNTEER COORDINATOR

	Exceeds	Meets	Does not meet
E			
P/S			
F			

(*E=employee, P/S=pastor/supervisor, F=final scoring)

Coordinates health ministry volunteer activity (may include student nurses or paid staff) by:

 a. recruiting volunteers for various health ministry activities

 b. providing orientation and continuing education for volunteers

 c. directing volunteer activities

 d. evaluating volunteer performance and providing appropriate feedback and recognition

Comments:

COLLEGIALITY

	Exceeds	Meets	Does not meet
E			
P/S			
F			

(*E=employee, P/S=pastor/supervisor, F=final scoring)

Maintains a positive working relationship with others by:

 a. participating in regular meeting with the parish pastor and staff

 b. meeting with and providing staff support for the health cabinet or advisory board

 c. actively participating in the parish nurse program meetings of the sponsoring organization (if applicable)

 d. participating in the wider local parish nurse network or other professional organizations

Comments:

EDUCATION

	Exceeds	Meets	Does not meet
E			
P/S			
F			

(*E=employee, P/S=pastor/supervisor, F=final scoring)

Acquires and maintains current knowledge in nursing practice, health promotion, and spiritual care by:

   a. participating in in-service programs and other educational activities authorized by the congregation/ministry

   b. attending any programs deemed mandatory by the sponsoring organization (if applicable)

Comments:

QUALITY ASSURANCE

	Exceeds	Meets	Does not meet
E			
P/S			
F			

(*E=employee, P/S=pastor/supervisor, F=final scoring)

Systematically participates in evaluation of quality and effectiveness of practice by:

   a. evaluating the ministries on a continuing basis with appropriate parties

   b. providing the congregation and (sponsoring organization) with appropriate statistical data in a timely fashion

c. participating in quality assurance activities initiated by the congregation and/or (sponsoring organization)

d. documenting services provided according to congregation and/or (sponsoring organization) requirements

Comments:

Goals and Accomplishments

Summarize goals established at (or since) the last review. Comment on actions taken to reach stated goals.

Summarize areas for improvement.

State any additional accomplishments since the last review date.

Clearly state goals for the next review period. Include personal and professional development plans as well as ways to enhance the ministries.

Parish nurse signature_____Date_____

Pastor/supervisor signature_____Date_____

Director of parish nursing signature_____Date_____

(Sponsoring organization, if applicable)_____

Appendix F

Parish Nurse Outcomes Measurement Tool

THE "PARISH NURSE OUTCOMES MEASUREMENT Tool" has been developed by Barbara Wehling, R.N., Ph.D., and Alvyne Rethemeyer, R.N., M.S.N., to address several questions that may be of interest to congregations and donors, including foundations and other grant makers. Those questions include the following:

1. Do parish nurses affect change in the health behaviors of those served?

2. Are parish nurses easily accessible to members of the congregation?

3. How are parish nurses serving the congregation and community?

4. How does the congregation respond to parish nurse programming?

5. What is the level of volunteer support for the program?

This survey can be ordered through the International Parish Nurse Resource Center. A congregation or parish nurse program orders the number of copies of the survey they think they will use. The cost per copy for the survey also includes the cost of data analysis and reporting.

Upon receipt of the completed surveys from a congregation or parish nurse program, the International Parish Nurse Resource Center will then tabulate the data and mail an Executive Summary and Report for use by the pastor, parish nurse, health cabinet, and congregation.

For more information on ordering copies of the survey, or to request a sample survey, please contact the International Parish Nurse

Resource Center at 314-918-2559, or visit the Web site at <www.parishnurses.org>.

Appendix G
Parish Nurse Resources

T HE FOLLOWING IS CERTAINLY NOT an exhaustive list of parish nurse resources, but these organizations are a good place to start.

International Parish Nurse Resource Center (IPNRC)
475 East Lockwood Avenue
St. Louis, Missouri 63119
Phone: 314-918-2559
Fax: 314-918-2558
E-mail: dpatterson@eden.edu
Web site: <www.parishnurses.org>

The IPNRC sponsors the annual Westberg Parish Nurse Symposium, maintains a parish nurse basic preparation curriculum in cooperation with educational partners around the United States and abroad, and provides parish nursing information and resources for congregations and parish nurse programs.

Health Ministries Association, Incorporated (HMA)
980 Canton Street
Bldg 1, Suite B
Roswell, GA 30075
Phone: 800-280-9919 or 770-640-9955
Fax 770-640-1095
E-mail: hmassoc@mindspring.com
Web site: <www.hmassoc.org>

This membership organization is for persons interested in health ministries, including clergy and chaplains, parish nurses, parish nurse program coordinators, educators, and lay health workers. HMA has local chapters and sponsors an annual conference. Developed the

Scope and Standards of Parish Nursing Practice, which was published in 1998 by American Nurses Publishing.

Interfaith Health Program
Rollins School of Public Health at Emory University
750 Commerce Street, Suite #301
Decatur GA 30030
Phone: 404-592-1461
Fax: 404-592-1462
Web site: <www.ihpnet.org>

The Interfaith Health Program assists in coordinating many different faith groups in their health outreach programs. This website has a large number of resources listed, from denominational contacts to health-related databases. IHP also publishes a newsletter and has an e-mail discussion list on faith and health issues.

Eden Bookstore
475 E. Lockwood Avenue
St. Louis, MO 63119
Phone: 877-627-5653 (toll-free) or 314-918-2500
Fax: 314-918-2520
E-mail: bookstore@eden.edu
Web site: <http://www.eden.edu/bookstore/bookstore.html>

Eden carries a wide selection of books and videos on parish nursing, as well as other books related to pastoral care and theology.

Mayo Foundation for Medical Education and Research
200 First Street S.W.
Rochester, MN 55905
Phone: 507-284-2511
Fax: 507-284-0161
Web site: <www.mayoclinic.org>

This foundation, associated with the Mayo Clinics, has an excellent Web site with health information <www.mayoclinic.com> and a free e-mail health bulletin that would provide excellent resources for parish nurse newsletter articles and bulletin boards.

Permission to reprint is free to parish nurses and congregations, and the Web site has directions on how to request permission to reprint by e-mail.

Centers for Disease Control and Prevention (CDC)
National Center for Health Statistics, Division of Data Services
Hyattsville, MD 20782-2003
Phone: 301-458-4636
Web site: <www.cdc.gov/nchs>

This government organization, part of the United States Department of Health and Human Services, provides a wide range of health data and information on health trends for use in parish nurse program planning.

United States Department of Health and Human Services
200 Independence Avenue, S.W.
Washington, D.C. 20201
Phone: 202-619-0257
Toll-free: 877-696-6775
Web site: <www.healthfinder.gov>

The Healthfinder® website provides a wealth of information on hundreds of diseases and health issues, which is easily accessible to the lay reader. It also includes a number of resources for promoting wellness and prevention, such as "on-line check-ups." The site has a databank on claims against doctors, hospitals, nursing homes, and health insurance companies and a carefully selected directory of other health-related Web sites.

American Public Health Association (APHA)
800 I Street, NW
Washington, DC 20001-3710
Phone: 202-777-APHA
Fax: 202-777-2534
Web site: <www.apha.org>

APHA's Web site has links to state public health associations and includes a number of resources for anyone interested in public health.

Healthy People 2010
Office of Disease Prevention and Health Promotion
Hubert H. Humphrey Building, Room 738G
200 Independence Avenue, SW
Washington, DC 20201
Phone: 202-205-2317
Fax: 202-205-9478
Web site: <www.healthypeople.gov>

Healthy People 2010 has developed a list of leading health indicators and goals for improvements in each of these areas by 2010. This is a good site to visit when planning parish nurse programming. The site also includes listings of current activities for implementation of improvements in each of these areas, which may be of interest to parish nurses.

Notes

Foreword

1. Names of those served have been changed.

Preface and Acknowlegements

1. Please see the resources listed at the end of this book for more information on these and other publications related to parish nursing and congregational health ministry.

2. Although the vast majority of parish nurses currently are women, increasing numbers of men are becoming interested and active in the field, and this great imbalance may change in the future.

3. Rev. Dr. Ellerbrake's description of the health-care system as "broken and dangerous" led to his conclusion that parish nursing is sorely needed in America today.

Chapter One

1. The Pope forbade clergy to shed blood in performance of surgery—hence the emergence of "barber-surgeons" with their red (blood) and white (bandages) poles. For more information, see link from the state of Tennessee's Web site at <http://www.state.tn.us/commerce/boards/barber/bpolehis.html>.

2. For more information on the Church and medicine, please read Jill Westberg McNamara's excellent chapter on medicine and the Christian Church in her book *The Health Cabinet: How to Start a Health Cabinet in Your Church* (1997; reprint, St. Louis: International Parish Nurse Resource Center, 2000); or refer to the work of Tom Droege in *The Theological Roots of Wholistic Health Care*, ed. Granger E. Westberg (Hinsdale, Ill.: Wholistic Health Centers, 1979).

3. Droege, in *Theological Roots*, 26.

4. The Evangelical Synod of North America is one of the predecessors of the United Church of Christ, a mainline Protestant denomination in the United States.

5. Romans 16:1–2.

6. See chapter 3, "Egypt, Greece, and Kaiserswerth," in Barbara Dossey, *Florence Nightingale: Mystic, Visionary, and Healer* (Springhouse, Pa.: Springhouse Publishing, 2000), 68–69, 74–78.

7.   For more information on the Deaconess Sisterhood and Deaconess Hospital in St. Louis, please see the book by Ruth Rasche, entitled *The Deaconess Heritage* (St. Louis: The Deaconess Foundation, 1994). Chapter 2 of the book, "The Deaconess Sisters, Pioneer Professional Women," which was also used in *Hidden Histories in the United Church of Christ*, edited by Barbara Brown Zikmund (New York: United Church Press, 1984) is available on the <www.parishnurses.org> Web site through a hyperlink in the "History" section about Deaconess Parish Nurse Ministries. The upper age limit of forty for admission to the Deaconess Sisterhood was waived for Sister Katherine Haack, a pastor's widow and the first Evangelical Sister in St. Louis, aged forty-nine. See Rasche, *Deaconess History*, 21.

8.   Mrs. Zipf was a board member of the Evangelical Deaconess Society and a member of an Evangelical congregation. She is a shining example of how health ministry can flourish, given the generosity of one or more individuals. See Rasche, *Deaconess History*, 7.

9.   For more information on health conditions in St. Louis at the time, see Rasche, *Deaconess History*, 2–4.

10. For more information on the Deaconess Foundation, see the Web site at <www.deaconess.org>.

11. "Problem of Lost Health Benefits is Reaching into the Middle Class," *The New York Times*, Monday, 25 November 2002.

Chapter Two

1.   Remark from an address given at the "Faith and Health Conference" sponsored by the Deaconess Foundation in St. Louis in 1999.

2.   Norbert Brox, "'Making Earth into Heaven': Diakonia in the Early Church," in Norbert Greinacher, Norbert Mette, and James Aitken Gardiner, eds., *Diakonia: Church for Others*, Concilium 198 (Edinburgh: T & T Clark, 1988), 33–40.

3.   For more information about diakonal ministry, see the book by James I. McCord and T. H. L. Parker, eds., *Service in Christ: Essays Presented to Karl Barth on his 80th Birthday* (Grand Rapids: William B. Eerdmans, 1966).

Chapter Three

1.   Taken from William M. Peterson, ed., *Granger Westberg Verbatim* (Hinsdale, Ill.: Westberg Institute, 1972), produced for the inaugural of the Westberg Institute. Reprinted in 2002 by the International Parish Nurse Resource Center, St. Louis, Missouri.

2.   See Granger E. Westberg, *The Parish Nurse: Providing a Minister of Health for Your Congregation* (Minneapolis: Augsburg Fortress, 1990).

3.   The International Parish Nurse Resource Center reprinted the 1997 edition in 2002.

4.   Unfortunately, the symposium began two days following the September 11 terrorism attack on the United States, and attendance was just over

four hundred, a remarkable commitment to this professional gathering of parish nurses, given the traumatic national circumstances at the time.

5. This book was subsequently published by Augsburg Fortress in 1990, the edition which remains available today.

6. This projection is based on the numbers of registered nurses who have completed the parish nurse basic preparation class developed by the IPNRC, adjusted for two factors: there are other parish nurse basic preparation curricula in use, and not every nurse becomes a parish nurse after taking the classes.

7. In 1997, parish nursing was recognized as a specialty by the American Nurses Association, and in 1998, the *Scope and Standards of Parish Nursing Practice*, which was developed by the Practice and Education Committee of the Health Ministries Association, acknowledged by the American Nurses Association, Congress of Nursing Practice, and published by American Nurses Publishing in Washington, D.C.

Chapter Four

1. The Faith in Action program was conceived in 1983 by the Robert Wood Johnson Foundation, which provides start-up grants for congregational programs working in partnership to improve the health of communities through volunteer interfaith caregiving. For more information, visit their Web site at <www.rwjf.org>.

Chapter Five

1. For more on the role of the health cabinet, we would refer you to Jill Westberg McNamara's excellent treatment on the topic, entitled *The Health Cabinet: How to Start A Wellness Committee in Your Church* (1997; reprint, St. Louis: International Parish Nurse Resource Center, 2002).

2. See McNamara, *The Health Cabinet*, and Granger E. Westberg and Jill Westberg McNamara, *The Parish Nurse: Providing a Minister of Health for Your Congregation* (Minneapolis: Augsburg Fortress, 1990).

Chapter Seven

1. Wendy RuthStiver et al. (Health Ministries Association), *Scope and Standards of Parish Nursing Practice* (Washington, D.C.: American Nurses Publishing, 1998) is available through the American Nurses Publishing House, 600 Maryland Avenue SW, Suite 100 West, Washington, DC 20024-2571, through the Health Ministries Association, Inc., 1930 Cedar Street, Ramona, CA 92065, or through the Eden Bookstore at 877-627-5653 (toll-free).

Chapter Eight

1. For more information, see Wendy RuthStiver et al. (Health Ministries Association), *Scope and Standards of Parish Nursing Practice* (Washington, D.C.: American Nurses Publishing, 1998) For more information on issues related to liability insurance, please see the chapter on providing benefits for a parish nurse.

Chapter Nine

1. These and other figures are in U.S. dollars and are based on costs in 2003 for a parish nurse in the St. Louis area of the Midwest. You will want to check other programs in your area to identify a competitive starting salary.

Chapter Ten

1. The Association of Fundraising Professionals (formerly the National Society of Fundraising Executives) also has many educational programs on fundraising fundamentals, many of which are open (for a slightly higher fee) to those who are not members. The association's Web site is <www.nsfre.org> and its address is 1101 King Street, Suite 700, Alexandria, VA 22314. Phone: 703-684-0410.

2. These and other figures are in U.S. dollars, and are based on costs in 2003 for a parish nurse in the St. Louis area of the Midwest.

3. Joy Skjegstad, chapter 10, "Successful Fundraising," in *Starting a Nonprofit at Your Church* (Bethesda, Md.: The Alban Institute, 2002), 132–47.

Chapter Eleven

1. The sample parish nurse job description in appendix A is one that fits within the Scope and Standards of Parish Nursing Practice as defined by the Health Ministries Association.

2. For more information on the Westberg Symposium, visit the Web site of the International Parish Nurse Resource Center, <www.parishnurses.org>.

3. For more information on the Health Ministries Association's annual conference, see appendix G, "Parish Nurse Resources."

Chapter Twelve

1. Educational Partners and the dates of the courses offered, with contact information, are listed at <www.parishnurses.org>.

Chapter Thirteen

1. Please see appendix B for a health needs assessment survey, which can be easily used within a congregational setting.

2. See appendix F for information on this Parish Nurse Outcomes Measurement Tool and chapter 14, "Parish Nurse Programming."

Appendix C

1. An anthem suitable for solo or unison choral or congregational singing, which was written for parish nurse installation and commissioning in St. Louis, is entitled "Your Hands Are God's Hands." It is available through the International Parish Nurse Resource Center.

2. This version of the doxology was published in *The Book of Worship, United Church of Christ* (New York: United Church of Christ Office for Church Life and Leadership, 1986), 66.

3. These lyrics to this well-known tune were written (unpublished until now) by the author, Rev. Deborah Patterson, in about 1996.

Bibliography

Baylor, Barbara. *Healthy Connections: A Compendium of UCC Congregational Ministries in Health, Welfare, and Human Service.* Cleveland: United Church of Christ, 2000.

Beard, Augustus Field. *The Story of John Frederic Oberlin.* Boston: Pilgrim Press, 1909.

Beckman, Richard J., and Steven Nerheim. *Toward a Healing Ministry: Exploring and Implementing a Congregational Ministry.* Minneapolis: Augsburg, 1985.

Carlson, Mim. *Winning Grants Step by Step: Support Centers of America's Complete Workbook for Planning, Developing and Writing Successful Proposals.* San Francisco: Jossey-Bass Publishers, 1995.

Carson, Verna Benner, and Harold G. Koenig. *Parish Nursing: Stories of Service and Care.* Radnor, Pa.: Templeton Foundation Press, 2002.

Claman, Victor N., and David E. Butler, with Jessica A. Boyatt. *Acting on Your Faith: Congregations Making a Difference.* Boston: Insights Inc., 1995.

Collins, John. *Diakonia: Reinterpreting the Ancient Sources.* New York: Oxford University Press, 1990.

Dossey, Barbara. *Florence Nightingale: Mystic, Visionary, and Healer.* Springhouse, Pa.: Springhouse Publishing, 2000.

Evans, Abigail Rian. *The Healing Church: Practical Programs for Health Ministries.* Cleveland: United Church Press, 1999.

Evans, Abigail Rian. *Redeeming Marketplace Medicine: A Theology of Health Care.* Cleveland: Pilgrim Press, 1999.

Golden, Susan L. *Successful Grantsmanship: A Guerilla Guide to Raising Money*. San Francisco: Jossey-Bass Publishers, 1997.

Greinacher, Norbert, Norbert Mette, and James Aitken Gardiner, eds. *Diakonia: Church for Others*. Concilium 198. Edinburgh: T. & T. Clark, 1988.

Gunderson, Gary. *Deeply Woven Roots: Improving the Quality of Life in Your Community*. Minneapolis: Augsburg Fortress, 1997.

Harley, Julie Ruth. *Soul Calling: Breathing Spirit into a Life of Service*. Cleveland: United Church Press, 1998.

Kenner, Carole, and Marlene Walden. *Grant Writing Tips for Nurses and Other Health Professionals*. Washington, D.C.: American Nurses Publishing, 2001.

Klein, Kim. *Ask and You Shall Receive: A Fund-raising Training Program for Religious Organizations and Projects, Participant Manual and Leader Manual*. San Francisco: Jossey-Bass Publishers, 2002.

Loomis, Evarts G., and J. Sig Paulson. *Healing for Everyone: Medicine of the Whole Person*. New York: Hawthorn Books, 1975.

Marty, Martin, and Kenneth L. Vaux, eds. *Health/Medicine and the Faith Traditions: An Inquiry into Religion and Medicine*. Philadelphia: Fortress Press, 1982.

McCord, James I., and T. H. L. Parker, eds. *Service in Christ: Essays Presented to Karl Barth on His 80th Birthday*. Grand Rapids: William B. Eerdmans, 1966.

McNamara, Jill Westberg. *The Health Cabinet: How to Start a Wellness Committee in Your Church*. 1997. Reprint, St. Louis: International Parish Nurse Resource Center, 2002.

McKee, Elsie Anne. *Diakonia in the Classical Reformed Tradition and Today*. Grand Rapids: William B. Eerdmans, 1989.

Mild, Mary L., ed. *Women at the Well: Meditations on Healing and Wholeness*. Valley Forge, Pa.: Judson Press, 1996.

Miller, Rev. Kent C. *Laying the Foundations: A Healing Presence . . .The Congregation's Ministry in Health and Wholeness.* San Antonio: Benedictine Resource Center, 1991.

Monchesky, Elenna, Elizabeth Schantz, and Henry Fischer. *Pioneers in Parish Nursing in Canada.* Toronto: University of Toronto, 1997.

Palmer, Parker. *The Active Life: A Spirituality of Work, Creativity and Caring.* New York: Harper Collins, 1990.

Peterson, William M., ed. *Granger Westberg Verbatim.* Hinsdale, Ill.: Westberg Institute, 1972.

Peterson, William M., ed. *Granger Westberg Verbatim: A Vision for Faith and Health.* St. Louis: International Parish Nurse Resource Center, 2002.

Rasche, Ruth. *The Deaconess Heritage.* St. Louis: The Deaconess Foundation, 1994.

RuthStiver, Wendy, et al. (Health Ministries Association). *Scope and Standards of Parish Nursing Practice.* Washington, D.C.: American Nurses Publishing, 1998.

Rosenberg, Charles. *The Care of Strangers.* New York: Basic Books, 1987.

Shields, Charles, and Cynthia Ferrell. *Spiritual Survival Guide: How to Find God When You're Sick.* New York: Doubleday, 2001.

Skjegstad, Joy. *Starting a Nonprofit at Your Church.* Bethesda, Md.: The Alban Institute, 2002.

Solari-Twadell, Phyllis Ann, and Mary Ann McDermott, eds. *Parish Nursing: Promoting Whole Person Health Within Faith Communities.* Thousand Oaks, Calif.: Sage Publications, 1999.

Starr, Paul. *The Social Transformation of American Medicine.* New York: Basic Books, 1982.

Vishnewskii, Stanley, ed. *Meditations: Dorothy Day.* New York: Harper and Row, 1952.

Wallis, Jim. *Faith Works: Lessons from the Life of an Activist Preacher.* New York: Random House, 2000.

Westberg, Granger E., and Jill Westberg McNamara. *The Parish Nurse: Providing a Minister of Health for Your Congregation.* Minneapolis: Augsburg Fortress, 1990.

Westberg, Granger E., ed. *Theological Roots of Wholistic Health Care.* Hinsdale, IL: Wholistic Health Centers, 1979.

Other books from The Pilgrim Press

The Healing Church
Practical Programs for Health Ministries
Abigail Rian Evans
ISBN 0-8298-1309-8/paper/260 pages/$24.00

What role can churches and religious organizations play in health care today? Abigail Rian Evans answers this question and others in this valuable guide to practical programs for health ministries. It includes a vast list of existing ministries that can be used as models.

Redeeming Marketplace Medicine
A Theology of Health Care
Abigail Rian Evans
ISBN 0-8298-1310-1/paper/208 pages/$17.00

Evans asserts that corporate-based managed care places profits over patient care. She further points out that medical experts have reduced health care to medical treatment under arrangements with health insurance plans and health maintenance organizations. Providing an engaging Christian theology, Evans proposes a broader health-care model.

Soul Calling
Breathing Life into a Life of Service
Julie Ruth Harley
ISBN 08298-1278-4/paper/144 pages/$16.00

Harley identifies difficulties presented by ministries that create stumbling blocks to spiritual growth. Writing in a personal meditative tone, Harley presents spiritually nourishing activities that will enable those in service ministries to develop their spiritual discipline—and deepen the sense of meaning in their lives and ministries.

Health as Liberation
Medicine, Theology, and the Quest for Justice
Alastair V. Campbell
ISBN 0-8298- 1022-6/cloth/112 pages /$15.00

In this lucid and moving analysis of what constitutes a theologically grounded understanding of authentic health care, ethicist Campbell relates the cases of those not often heard—those vulnerable patients in hospital wards. He demonstrates convincingly why all of us—both inside and outside of Washington—need to listen.

Medicine as Ministry
Reflections on Suffering, Ethics, and Hope
Margaret E. Mohrmann, M.D.
ISBN 0-8298-1073-0/paper/120 pages/$13.00

How does one begin to reconcile faith in a merciful God with the crushing reality of human suffering? For twenty years, Mohrmann has sought to heal children racked by disease and dysfunction, helping many to recover—and watching some die. This book is her moving story of the implications of a theological understanding of health, illness, and hope.

Pain Seeking Understanding
Suffering, Medicine, and Faith
Margaret E. Mohrmann and Mark J. Hanson, editors
ISBN 0-8298-1354-3/paper/224 pages/$2.30 net

This resource examines how believers and nonbelievers alike wrestle with questions of faith when confronted with pain and suffering that medicine alone cannot treat. Fellow experts in the fields of medicine, ethics, theology, and pastoral care help to weave the complex story of faith and science.

To order these or any other books from The Pilgrim Press, call or write to:

The Pilgrim Press
700 Prospect Avenue East
Cleveland, Ohio 44115-1100

Phone orders: 800-537-3394 • Fax orders: 216-736-2206
Please include shipping charges of $4.00 for the first book and $0.75 for each additional book.
Or order from our Web sites at <www.pilgrimpress.com> and <www.unitedchurchpress.com>.

Prices subject to change without notice.